Application of Manufacturers' Sound Data

This publication was prepared under ASHRAE Research Project 786 by Scantek, Inc., Silver Spring, Maryland. It was sponsored by TC 2.6, Sound and Vibration Control.

About the Authors:

Charles Ebbing *is a senior staff acoustical engineer at Carrier Corp. with over 31 years of experience as an acoustical consultant. He is the recipient of the 1991 ARI Schulze Distinguished Service Award for Leadership in Acoustical Standards and the 1994 ASHRAE TC 2.6 Outstanding Service Award. He is an active member of ASHRAE TC 2.6 and serves on the ARI Technical Committee on Sound.*

Warren Blazier *is president of Warren Blazier Associates, a consulting firm specializing in HVAC acoustics, noise, and vibration control. He is a Fellow and Life Member of ASHRAE and the recipient of several awards. Among these are Best State of the Art Technical Paper—1972, 1981; Crosby Field Award for Best Paper of Outstanding Quality—1972, 1981.*

Ted Carnes *is a registered professional mechanical engineer with over 20 years of experience as an acoustical consultant. He is a senior consultant in Dallas at Pelton Marsh Kinsella, which is the acoustical consulting division of Carter & Burgess. He is an active member of ASHRAE TC 2.6.*

Brian Guenther *is president of Vibro-Acoustics, a manufacturer specializing in noise control for fans and air-handling units. He is publications chair of ASHRAE TC 2.6 and a member of ASTM Committee E-33 on Environmental Acoustics. He is the editor for the 1999 ASHRAE Handbook—Applications chapter, "Sound and Vibration Control."*

Tom Paige *is a senior engineer and marketing manager with Vibron Limited, a wholly owned subsidiary of Kinetics Noise Control, Inc. He has over ten years of experience in acoustical engineering and has presented and published many technical papers on case studies involving HVAC noise and vibration control.*

John Paulauskis *is an acoustical engineer at HBE Corporation with over 24 years of experience as an acoustical engineer and consultant. He is a member of ASHRAE and the Institute of Noise Control Engineers.*

Raymond Vanderburgh *is retired from Vibro-Acoustics where he was the senior research and development engineer and technical advisor. He is an INCE member and past member of ASHRAE TC 2.6. He has over 20 years of experience in noise control application engineering, product design and development, acoustic laboratory design, and laboratory and field testing of silencers, acoustic panels, compartment and custom ultra-quiet air-handling units, and design of low-energy duct systems.*

Application of Manufacturers' Sound Data

Edited by Charles Ebbing and Warren Blazier

American Society of Heating, Refrigerating
and Air-Conditioning Engineers, Inc.

ISBN 1-883413-62-1

1791 Tullie Circle N.E.
Atlanta, Georgia 30329
www.ashrae.org

Printed in the United States of America

Cover illustration by Rodney A. Mays

ASHRAE Staff

SPECIAL PUBLICATIONS

Mildred Geshwiler
Editor
Jeri Alger
Managing Editor
Jennifer Schonheiter
Assistant Editor
Amanda Arwood
Assistant Editor
Michshell Phillips
Secretary

PUBLISHING SERVICES

Scott Zeh
Manager
Jayne Jackson
Production Assistant

PUBLISHER

W. Stephen Comstock

Table of Contents

Chapter 4—Fan Noise Characteristics Tutorial

Chapter 5—Central-Station Air-Handling Units

Chapter 6—Commercial Packaged HVAC Equipment

Chapter 7—Silencers for HVAC Systems

CHAPTER 12—ROOM FAN COIL UNITS

CHAPTER 13—CENTRIFUGAL WATER PUMPS

CHAPTER 14—AIR-COOLED CHILLERS AND CONDENSING UNITS

CHAPTER 15—WATER-COOLED CHILLERS

CHAPTER 16—COOLING TOWERS

CHAPTER 17—OVERVIEW OF HVAC TEST PROCEDURES

Preface

About a decade ago, members of ASHRAE TC 2.6, Sound and Vibration Control, recognized that one of its primary functions was to facilitate the generation of quality, up-to-date acoustical information in a practical format for use by the ASHRAE membership. The publication of the first book sponsored by TC 2.6, *A Practical Guide to Noise and Vibration Control for HVAC Systems*, was well received by the Society. As a result, the committee decided to sponsor this second guide that focuses on improving the understanding and appropriate use of manufacturers' acoustical data. This book is the result of ASHRAE Research Project 786.

The main purpose of this book is to clarify how HVAC manufacturers' acoustical data and application information can best be used. The book is intended to provide a better understanding of the following factors important in the design and application process:

- Industry sound standards
- Testing and rating procedures
- Typical assumptions that are made when obtaining or applying acoustical test data
- System design issues that should be considered
- Application issues that should be considered

It is assumed that the principal users of this book will be mechanical engineers, acoustical consultants, system designers, contractors, building owners, manufacturers, and others concerned with the specification and commissioning of building systems, as well as those persons troubleshooting after-the-fact HVAC-related noise problems.

Noise problems cannot be avoided by depending entirely upon manufacturers' data and application guidelines. Good system design practices are also necessary to avoid unanticipated noise problems. Designers need to be aware that, even with all the analytical factors taken into account, it is only by the judicious use of manufacturers' data and application guidelines, together with good system design practices, that system noise problems can be avoided.

Charles Ebbing and Warren Blazier
Editors

Acknowledgments

The information in this book was taken from many sources and was produced with the help of many people. The authors and editors would like to express their special appreciation to the following people:

Members of the ASHRAE Monitoring Committee for this project (RP-786):

- Mr. William Fearon (Chair)
- Dr. Ted Carnes
- Mr. Robert Hoover
- Mr. Mark Schaffer
- Mr. Ray Vanderburgh
- Dr. Alf Warnock

Mr. Robert Harold for his efforts in proposing and gaining acceptance for this research project.

Mr. Daniel Fragnito for his assistance in reviewing Chapters 4 and 5.

Mr. Dan Int-Hout for his assistance in preparing Chapters 10 and 11.

Mr. Robert Hoover, Mr. William Osborn, and Mr. Robert Miller for their assistance in reviewing Chapter 16.

Mr. Dennison Chamberlain for his encouragement and support of this effort.

Chapter 1
Using Manufacturers' Acoustical Data

by *Warren Blazier, Ted Carnes, Charles Ebbing, and John Paulauskis*

BOOK OVERVIEW

WHO THIS BOOK IS FOR

It is assumed that the primary readers of this book are mechanical engineers, acoustical consultants, designers, contractors, building owners, manufacturers, and others involved in the specification, design, sales, commissioning of buildings, and troubleshooting of HVAC-related building noise problems.

PURPOSE OF THIS BOOK

The purpose of this book is to help interpret and clarify how users can make the best use of HVAC manufacturers' acoustical data and application information. This book is intended to provide a better understanding of the following factors that are important in the design and application process:

- Typical assumptions that are made when obtaining or applying factory acoustical test data
- System design issues that should be considered
- Application issues that should be considered
- Industry acoustical measurement and rating standards
- Testing procedures

Noise problems cannot be avoided by depending entirely on manufacturers' data and application guidelines. Good system design practices are necessary to avoid noise problems. Designers also need to be aware that even with all the analytical factors taken into account, it is only by the judicious use of manufacturers' data and application guidelines, together with good system design practices, that noise problems can be avoided.

HVAC acoustical problems can be minimized by:

- Understanding the basis of manufacturers acoustical data
- Understanding how the project application may differ from that rated by the manufacturer
- Exercising good system design considerations

This book will also help in writing better acoustical specifications and give a better sense as to how to realistically use manufacturers' acoustical data. It is also useful in understanding and rectifying building noise problems involving commercial HVAC products.

BOOK ORGANIZATION

The chapters in this book are arranged by categories of HVAC equipment noise sources. This should permit the reader to rapidly locate information pertaining to a specific product type. While this may lead to some redundancy because certain information and application guidelines are common to several chapters, it is believed that this approach will make the book more flexible for the reader who simply wants to use it as a handbook.

HOW USEFUL IS MANUFACTURERS' ACOUSTICAL DATA?

When purchasing a new car, few of us expect to achieve the miles per gallon shown on the Environmental Protection Agency (EPA) sticker since the test conditions used to obtain this rating are different from the way we will drive the car. However, the ratings are useful in comparing the performance of several vehicles that we may consider for purchase. In a similar manner, the acoustical ratings of most HVAC products are useful for the comparison of competitive products under standardized conditions but are less meaningful for estimating acoustical performance in installed systems. By necessity, manufacturers cannot test products in all applications but must limit testing to the standardized conditions specified by the applicable test standard[1]. The remainder of this chapter briefly reviews the problems that affect manufacturers' acoustical data.

1. See Chapter 17, Table 17-1.

When Using Manufacturers' Data, Keep In Mind:

- Differences between lab test conditions and real applications
- Limitations of estimated data vs. measured data
- Manufacturers' difficulties in keeping sound data current
- Manufacturers' data may not cover what you want
- Sound power and sound pressure data are often confused
- Structureborne noise effects are often ignored in system design
- Tested equipment is usually in perfect condition, which results in optimistic ratings
- Even with good quality control, not all products are identical
- System effects are usually present in field applications
- Differences in interpretation of test standards by test labs

WHAT IS THE PROBLEM?

Lab Conditions vs. Field Applications

While many of the Air Conditioning and Refrigeration Institute (ARI) and Air Movement and Control Association (AMCA) sound ratings covered in this book are useful for comparing products tested under the same laboratory conditions, seldom do these ratings correspond to actual jobsite conditions. The failure to recognize these differences when determining product noise specifications is often the cause of unanticipated noise problems in the field.

The way HVAC components are assembled into a system affects the noise level. Too many engineers believe that satisfactory noise levels in occupied spaces can be achieved by simply using a manufacturer's sound ratings as a design tool without consideration of the system influence. Engineers need to realize that manufacturers can only provide products that meet a specification based on data obtained under standard conditions.

Limitations of Estimated Data

Manufacturers often use mathematical calculations, based on physical principles or test data, to estimate sound data on the non-tested products.

Some manufacturers use simplified computer programs and previously published ASHRAE (American Society of Heating, Refrigerating and Air-Conditioning Engineers, Inc.) fan equations no longer supported by ASHRAE to estimate product acoustical data. Many times sound estimation equations for fans and other HVAC equipment are derived from idealistic assumptions and often are of limited value in rating the actual equipment.

The interpolation or extrapolation of test data from one size unit to another, if not done with caution, can produce unreliable data. For example, larger fan diameters, slight changes in the rotational speed of driven components, different compressors, etc., can create significant differences in product sound emissions. Overlooking the contribution of auxiliary items required to make the product function may contribute to or reduce the product noise in an application and can introduce significant error in the noise estimation procedure.

Sound Data is Not Always Current

Maintaining current sound data for new equipment is a difficult task for HVAC manufacturers. Furthermore, because of the amount of testing involved to rate a product line, seldom is the data based on a large statistical sampling of the particular product being tested. Often, only a single sample of the product is tested, and this may be a prototype and not a production unit.

Manufacturers' Data May Not Cover Everything Desired

In many cases, the acoustical data available from a manufacturer may not cover the complete sound frequency range of interest, or the data may not be available at the specific system operating point or conditions desired.

Because ISO (International Organization for Standardization) and ANSI (American National Standards Institute) test standards do not address very low frequencies, very little to no industry data is published below 100 Hz. Although many fan manufacturers do publish data below 100 Hz, in some instances this may be subject to question because of the use of an inappropriate reference sound source or because the physical size of the acoustical test facility is too small to obtain valid low-frequency data. Furthermore, the available acoustical data is generally only for components, yet the designer may need to estimate system noise levels with reference to a specific noise criterion assigned a given space. This frequently establishes the need for data pertaining to the 63 Hz and 31.5 Hz octave bands. Much testing within this frequency region is performed in good faith, but not with a good understanding of the problems encountered in obtaining valid low-frequency data. Therefore, it is always advisable to inquire of the manufacturer as to the sound test procedure utilized, the rating procedure used, and the current status of any rating certification program on the equipment.

Manufacturers often publish only single number rating data, such as those expressed in dB(A), sones, or bels. For the noise control design of a field application, this type of rating information is entirely inadequate to describe the sound emitted by HVAC equipment. Therefore, it is incumbent on the designer to insist upon receiving adequate information concerning the complete frequency spectrum of the sound produced by the product. This book will help to bridge the gap between the sound ratings of individual system components and how these are used in an analysis of the overall system design.

Certain aspects of some testing and rating standards are written loosely enough to permit significantly different interpretations by different laboratories. As a result, the same product could achieve significantly different results in different laboratories. This potential error is included in the "Measurement Uncertainty of Standard Test Procedure" values that are in the appropriate table for each equipment type.

Sound Power and Sound Pressure are Often Confused

Sound data for some of the larger HVAC equipment, such as water-cooled chillers and cooling towers, are customarily presented in terms of sound pressure level at some specified distance from the product. Data for most other HVAC equipment are usually presented in terms of sound power level. It is very important to understand the differences between these two descriptors. Chapter 2 should clarify these differences for the reader.

Structureborne Noise

Many HVAC noise problems involve not only airborne sound, but also structureborne sound transmission. The control of structureborne noise involves vibration isolation of the mechanical equipment. This is discussed in each chapter of the book pertaining to a specific type of HVAC equipment where mechanical vibration can have a significant influence.

Manufacturers Usually Test Units in Perfect Operating Condition

Manufacturers' published data are seldom based upon a large statistical sampling of the product. Only a few units are normally tested, and these are usually in optimum condition at the time of testing. When a product is tested for sound by the manufacturer, great pains are usually taken to ensure that the unit is in the best physical condition possible. Typically, the laboratory personnel will generally determine the following:

1. The unit is assembled properly per specifications;
2. It has the proper refrigerant charge;
3. It is operated at specified operating conditions;
4. It has a clean aerodynamic configuration in the attachment of ductwork;
5. Screws and bolts are properly installed and tightened;
6. Fans and compressors are properly installed;
7. Refrigerant discharge and suction lines are properly clamped;
8. Vibration isolation is not bypassed or short circuited.

Deviation from any of these conditions in the field can increase the noise level of the product above the levels anticipated on the basis of the manufacturer's published data.

Variability Due to Manufacturing Quality Control

It is unrealistic to expect that a unit, which has been randomly selected from a production run and tested in the laboratory without modification(s) or adjustment(s), will precisely duplicate the published sound rating data. Most differences are likely attributable to production quality control.

External System Effects

The user should also be aware that sound data provided by most manufacturers are obtained under standardized laboratory test conditions. If the equipment is installed in a manner that differs from the test configuration, external system effects caused by a different configuration of connected ductwork, and interactions with other components of the installation, often significantly increase the operating noise level. For example, it is rare to find aerodynamically clean fan inlet and outlet conditions in the typical field application. Furthermore, components such as silencers are frequently installed in locations too close to the fan equipment for a uniform velocity profile to exist at the entrance to the silencer. This results in a significantly higher than anticipated pressure drop across that component. The combination of these two system effects changes the operating point on the fan curve, resulting in a reduction in airflow that must be compensated for by increasing the fan speed, with a substantial increase in noise.

The user needs to be constantly aware of the physical differences between field and laboratory test conditions and know the strengths and limitations of the test data when used in a specific application. A common trap many users fail to recognize is that the system installation configuration may differ significantly from that used by the manufacturer in the setup for testing. It must be recognized that the manufacturer cannot second-guess the variety of installation configurations that the product may encounter in field applications, and, thus, they cannot be held accountable for system effects not present in the standardized test setup used for performance rating.

Unfortunately, system effects are neglected in most currently available noise prediction methods. These estimation schemes typically assume that good design practices have been used in laying out the HVAC system. For example, the *1995 ASHRAE Handbook—Applications* (ASHRAE 1995) gives requirements for placement of elbows downstream of a fan discharge to minimize system effects, and guidelines for other elements of system design are provided in ASHRAE and SMACNA (Sheet Metal and Air Conditioning Contractors National Association, Inc.) publications (ASHRAE SMACNA 1981, 1985; Schaffer 1991). However, in both the design and installation of systems, where available space is frequently restricted and construction cost is a prime consideration, these guidelines are frequently not followed. Thus, noise estimation techniques that do not account for actual divergence from good design and installation practice inevitably lead to erroneous conclusions about the adequacy of system acoustical design.

Neglecting the influence of external system effects in the application of manufacturers' acoustical data can typically lead to the underprediction of noise levels by 5 dB to 15 dB, depending upon the particular circumstances of a given installation.

CUMULATIVE ERRORS

It is not likely that the potential cumulative error associated with the variability of data among laboratories, the variability associated with manufacturing prototype testing and quality control, and the variability due to external system effects in product application will "stack up" in a linear manner. Instead, it is more probable that the cumulative effect will be a random statistical mix of these variables, depending upon the circumstances associated with a particular system design and installation practice. In general, even if the best system design and installation practices are followed to minimize external system effects, a noise estimation model based upon manufacturers' published data will usually underpredict the result by at least 5 dB. However, if external effects are not minimized in system design and installation practices, the underprediction of overall system acoustical performance could easily approach 10 dB to 15 dB.

The excess system-generated noise can be manifested in several ways. It may be a low-frequency rumble radiated from fan-connected ductwork; a mid-frequency roar radiated through the ceiling of overhead air terminal valves and mixing boxes; a high frequency hiss from grilles, registers, and diffusers; or a combination of all three. While it may be fair to blame some of the uncertainty in noise estimation on the present quality of manufacturers' data, in the bigger picture it is clear that ignoring the influence of external system effects in design and installation practices is at least equally to blame. It is also fair to comment that cost-cutting decisions are frequently made without the benefit of input from persons who can comment objectively on the acoustical implications of a proposed change.

VALUE OF SOUND CERTIFICATION PROGRAMS

Sound certification programs have begun to emerge because of the growing pressures to reduce the uncertainties in manufacturers' sound data and to improve reliability in the estimation of acoustical performance in field installations. For example, in 1981, Blazier, under contract with ARI, conducted an independent audit of the quality of existing published data on air terminal devices of similar capacity being produced by seven leading manufacturers (Blazier 1981). His study revealed that there was poor agreement between published data and the actual performance measured independently

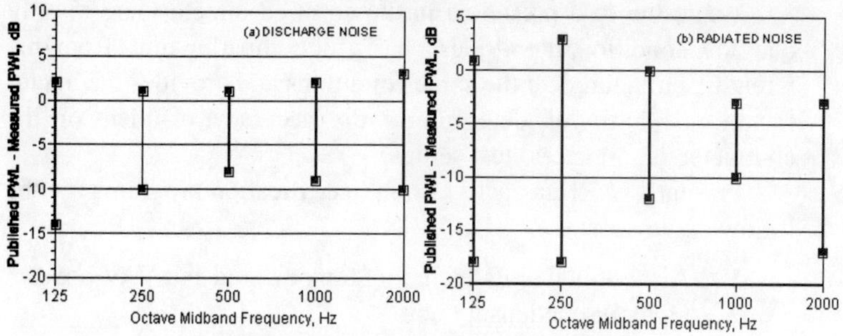

FIGURE 1-1 Range between measured and published sound power levels (PWL) of VAV terminals in a survey of seven manufacturers: (a) discharge noise, (b) radiated noise. Positive values indicate that the measured values were higher than those cataloged.

in supervised laboratory tests. The results of this audit are summarized in Figure 1-1. The illustration shows the range of variation between measured and published data found among the seven manufacturers in the survey; positive values indicate that the measured data were higher than those cataloged.

Upon completion of this study, ARI adopted a sound certification program for air terminal devices. Included in this program was the creation of a new method of test (ARI 880) that refined the previous test methods.

In this program, tests on random samples of production units are conducted by an independent acoustical laboratory to verify that sound levels do not exceed published ratings by more than a specified tolerance, as shown in Table 1-1.

TABLE 1-1
ARI 880 Tolerances

Octave Band (Hz)	125	250	500	1000	2000	4000
ARI 880 Tolerance	6 dB	5 dB	4 dB	3 dB	3 dB	3 dB

ARI 880-OM (Operations Manual) allows the tolerances in each octave band as indicated, plus 2 dB in one band, or plus 1 dB in two bands. Exceeding these limits results in a failure that requires that all other units of the same type be adjusted by the same number of dB as the difference between the listed value and the measured value in each band as part of the penalty. In addition, additional tests on other units, as well as on the unit that failed, are required the following year as part of the penalty.

While the data presented in the certified directory are at only one flow condition, it provides a basis for comparing units from different manufacturers at the same conditions and provides the manufacturers a basis of determining the accuracy of their or the contracted laboratories' test setups.

Presently, ARI has active sound certification programs for the following devices:

1. Air terminal units including fan powered and VAV boxes
2. Outdoor condensing units
3. Room fan-coil units

Since the initiation of the ARI program for terminal units, testing has refined the procedures (most recently ARI 880-1994 and an accompanying Operations Manual, ARI 880-OM), and most major manufacturers are now participants of the program. *Results of annual tests are evident in the directory, where a trend of fewer check test failures is becoming evident.*

AMCA sponsors a sound ratings certification program for fans that is also voluntary. An AMCA Certified Sound Ratings Seal can be obtained on fan equipment that has been independently tested under AMCA supervision at the AMCA laboratory. Periodic retesting for verification of ratings is required under the AMCA program; sound levels must be within the tolerances permitted by AMCA.

REFERENCES

ASHRAE. 1995. *1995 ASHRAE handbook—Applications*, pp. 43.21, 43.9. Atlanta: American Society of Heating, Refrigerating and Air-Conditioning Engineers, Inc.

Schaffer, M.E. 1991. *A practical guide to noise and vibration control for HVAC systems.* Atlanta: American Society of Heating, Refrigerating and Air-Conditioning Engineers, Inc.

SMACNA. 1981. *HVAC duct system design*, 2d ed. Vienna, Va: Sheet Metal and Air-Conditioning Contractors' Association.

SMACNA. 1985. *HVAC duct construction standards.* Vienna, Va: Sheet Metal and Air-Conditioning Contractors' Association.

Blazier, W.E. 1981. Noise rating of variable-air-volume terminal devices. *ASHRAE Transactions* 87(1): 140-152.

Chapter 2
Sound Power Level and Sound Pressure Level

by *Charles Ebbing, Warren Blazier*

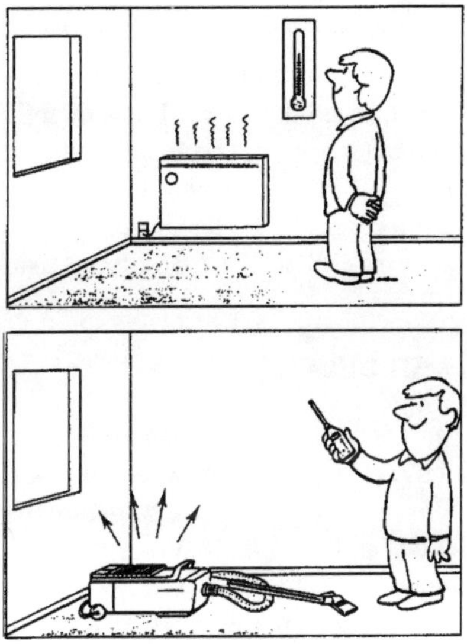

FIGURE 2-1 Sound analogy with heat.

THE DIFFERENCE BETWEEN SOUND POWER LEVEL (L_W) AND SOUND PRESSURE LEVEL (L_P) AS A BASIS FOR NOISE RATING

SOUND PRESSURE LEVEL (L_P)

What the human ear responds to and perceives as sound is the result of tiny pressure fluctuations above and below the static value of atmospheric pressure. These dynamic pressure fluctuations (force per unit area) cause the eardrum to vibrate, which begins a chain of events in the hearing process that result in signals the brain recognizes as sound. Thus, the quantity of interest, when describing the magnitude of sound perceived by the human ear, is the sound pressure.

The range of sound pressures corresponding to hearing sensations extending from very faint to very loud is too huge to measure on a linear scale. A logarithmic or decibel scale is used to compress the range into something manageable. Fortunately, the human ear is not a linear device but responds in a somewhat logarithmic way. Therefore, the use of the decibel scale (dB) is a convenient means of expressing the level of a given sound pressure with respect to a reference sound pressure of 2×10^{-5} Pa, corresponding to the threshold of human perception. Thus, the term sound pressure level (L_p) with respect to 2×10^{-5} Pa, is used as a descriptor of the sound environment as perceived by the human ear. It is a quantity that depends on the acoustical characteristics of the space, subject to many variables such as room size and geometry, and the amount and placement of acoustical absorption present in the space.

Sound pressure level is the quantity measured with a sound level meter.

SOUND POWER LEVEL (L_W)

A fundamental characteristic of an acoustic source is its ability to radiate sound power, whether weak and small in size (as a cricket) or strong and large (as a compressor). An energy input excites the source, and it radiates this energy in acoustical form. This acoustical power can be expressed in watts. Thus, *sound power* is the rate at which sound energy is radiated by a sound source. It is a property of the noise source, and the magnitude of power radiated by a given source is considered to be essentially independent of the surrounding environment. For this reason, it has become customary in the industry to express the acoustical properties of equipment in terms of the sound power output.[1]

The sound power of a source is determined from either mea-

1. Strictly speaking, there are special circumstances under which the sound power output of a device, especially at low frequencies, may be modified by the acoustical properties of the test environment. These effects are being investigated at the present time because of the increasing attention being paid to equipment noise characteristics in the frequency range below 100 Hz.

surements of sound pressure levels or by comparison to a source of known sound power (reference sound source). In some cases, the sound power of sources are estimated from calculations.

The range of sound power outputs from very quiet to the very loud sources of noise is too huge to handle on a linear scale, so again a logarithmic scale expressed in decibels (dB) is used to compress the range to something manageable. The decibel scale (dB) in this case is used as a means for expressing the level of a given sound power with respect to a reference sound power. The reference sound power typically used is 10^{-12} watt. Sound power level (L_w), with respect to 10^{-12} watt, is the common descriptor used by industry to express the sound power output of a piece of equipment.

The Differences Between L_W and L_P are Frequently Confusing

The fact that both the sound power level (L_w) and sound pressure level (L_p) are expressed in decibels creates much confusion in the engineering design of HVAC systems and the sound specifications of components. What is not understood is that a decibel is simply a means of expressing the magnitude of a specific quantity with respect to a reference quantity when the range of values involved is very large. For example, one could express the number of apples in a bushel as so many dB above a reference value of one apple. Often overlooked is the kind of reference quantity specified. The reference for sound power level is a power expressed in watts; the reference for sound pressure level is a pressure expressed as a force per unit area or pascal.

There is also confusion when applying L_w and L_p. It may help to consider the following analogy between sound and heat. The sound power of a source corresponds to the heat output of a source in Btu/h. Both depend only upon source characteristics. The sound pressure level corresponds to the temperature in the room. Both depend upon space and room properties that vary from space to space. This analogy is often helpful in understanding the difference between L_w and L_p, as illustrated in Figure 2-1.

There is also an analogy between sound and light. For example, the rate of energy consumption of a light bulb is expressed in watts, but the illumination produced in a given room depends upon the room size and the reflectivity of the surfaces. In the case of sound, the rate at which the source delivers energy to the space is expressed in watts, but the sound pressure level that results depends on the room size and the amount of acoustical absorption present.

SOUND PROPAGATION OUTDOORS

Outdoors, there are few reflecting surfaces aside from the ground. As a result, the sound pressure, due to the spherical propagation pattern of sound energy, typically decreases inversely as the square of the distance from the source to the receiver (Beranek 1971). As a result, sound level decreases with increasing distance between the noise source and sound receiver (Beranek 1971).

Figure 2-2 illustrates the relationship between the source sound power level, L_w, outdoors and the sound pressure level, L_p, at a given distance from the source. The L_p can be estimated at various locations by subtracting the path losses, such as might be introduced by barrier objects, and the loss due to spherical spreading. Appropriate factors to use are described in the *1995 ASHRAE Handbook* (ASHRAE 1995) and in various industry application standards (ARI 1984; ASHRAE 1991).

FREE AND REVERBERANT FIELDS

Free Field

A free field is one with no sound reflections. A source of sound located in a free-field environment produces a sound pressure level pattern changing only as a function of distance, due to only direct radiation from the source with no contributions due to reflected energy.

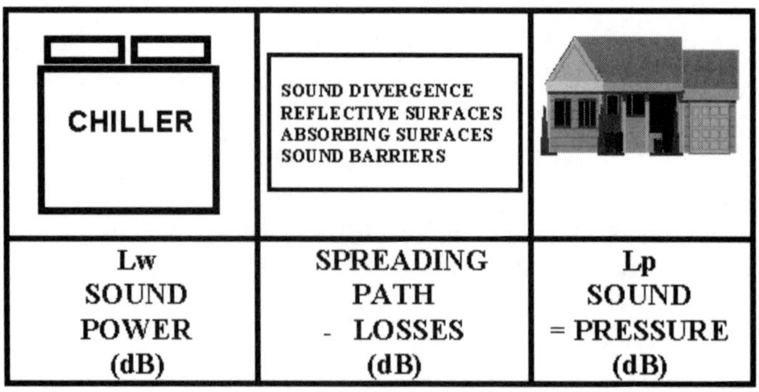

FIGURE 2-2 Relationship of sound power to sound pressure outdoors.

Essentially Free Field

Many times manufacturers' measured sound pressure level data, such as for cooling towers and water-cooled chillers and centrifugal pumps, are obtained under "essentially free-field conditions." A flat, open space with minimal obstructions except for the ground, or a very large volume room free of significant reflections, is often used to obtain essentially free-field sound data so that sound pressure levels close to the sound source are not affected by reflections from distant surfaces.

REVERBERANT FIELD

A reverberant field environment is one in which the magnitude of the sound pressure level in the space of interest is dominated by reflected sound energy. For example, a small mechanical equipment room with hard reflective surfaces is highly reverberant.

SOUND PROPAGATION INDOORS

Figure 2-3 illustrates the indoor relationship between sound power level, L_w, and sound pressure level, L_p. The estimation of sound pressure levels indoors is usually more complicated than in an outdoor situation because both the direct and reflected components of the sound energy have to be taken into account. In outdoor situations, usually only the direct sound component has to be estimated at the location of interest.

The sound pressure level indoors (at a specific location) can be estimated by subtracting from the known sound power level, L_w, the

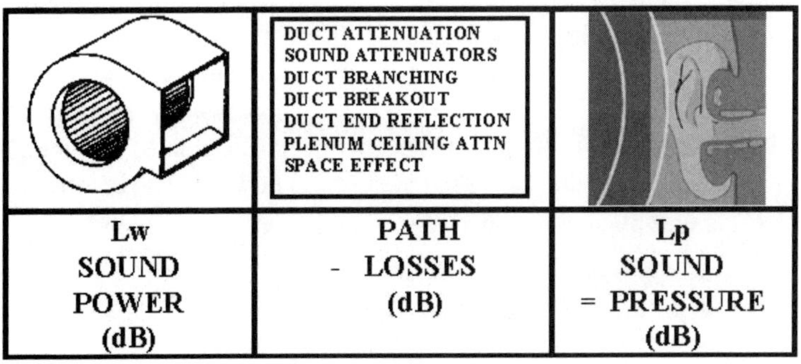

FIGURE 2-3 Relationship of sound power to sound pressure indoors.

energy losses that occur in the various sound paths between the sources and receiver. These losses in decibels are described in detail in the *ASHRAE Handbook* (ASHRAE 1995) and in various industry application standards (ARI 1990).

MOST SOURCES ARE RATED IN TERMS OF SOUND POWER LEVEL EXCEPT FOR COOLING TOWERS AND WATER-COOLED CHILLERS

While most HVAC sources are rated in terms of sound power level, cooling towers and water-cooled chillers are exceptions. These are rated in terms of sound pressure level measured at a specified distance from the face of the unit in essentially free-field conditions as previously described in this chapter.

Both ARI and the Cooling Tower Institute (CTI) recognize that very large equipment[2] is nearly impossible to rate unless the testing is accomplished in situ when the equipment is delivering rated tonnage. It is unrealistic to expect that these machines can be moved to a reverberant or anechoic space for testing. Consequently, these units are normally tested outdoors or in an essentially free-field environment indoors.

HOW SOUND PRESSURE LEVELS ARE ESTIMATED FROM SOUND POWER LEVELS (FAN POWERED TERMINAL EXAMPLE)

Figure 2-4 (after ARI Standard 885-90) illustrates the acoustical model of a fan-powered air terminal device. This model shows six paths that the sound can take to reach the receiver's ears. Most often, only one or two of the paths are significant contributors, which can simplify the calculations. In most cases, paths 1 and 5 are usually the most significant contributors to the receiver's sound level.

- For Path 1, the sound pressure level is calculated by subtracting from the casing radiated sound power level (L_w) the ceiling-plenum attenuation (P) and the space effect (S).

2. Cooling towers are usually tested at 5 ft and 50 ft from the source. Water-cooled chillers are tested at 1 m from the chiller surfaces at a height of 1.5 m above the floor. Cooling towers and water-cooled chillers are rated in terms of sound pressure level at specified distances from the source.

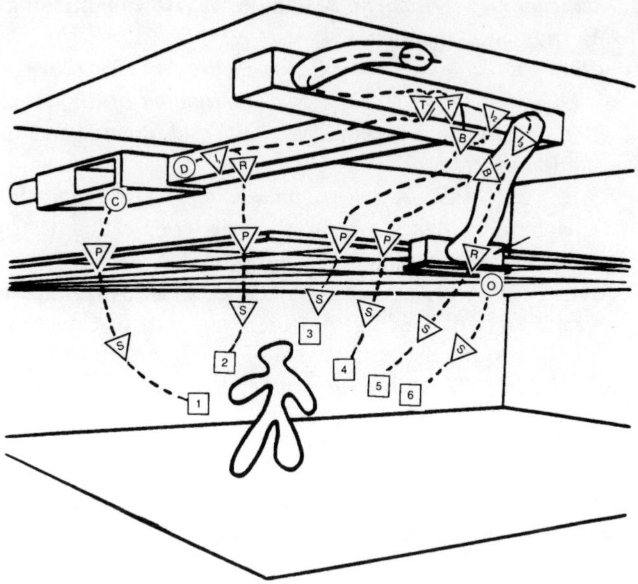

Path 1- sound breakout from the casing of the unit
Path 2- sound breakout from the discharge duct
Path 3- sound breakout from follow-on ducting
Path 4- sound breakout from flexible ducting
Path 5- discharge sound radiating to the room through the entire duct system, openings, etc.
Path 6- airflow generated noise from the outlet

FIGURE 2-4 Sound paths from noise sources to receiver in occupied space from ARI 880.

- For Path 5, the sound pressure level is calculated by subtracting from the discharge sound power level (*D*) the duct insertion losses, elbow and tee losses, branch power division, end reflection factor, and the space effect (*S*).
- These two sound pressure levels are then added logarithmically to estimate the sound pressure level for the octave band of interest.
- For critical applications, the sound pressure level of all paths should be added logarithmically.

REFERENCES

ARI. 1984. *ARI Standard 275-84, Application of sound rated out-*

door unitary equipment. Arlington, Va: Air Conditioning and Refrigeration Institute.

ARI. 1990. *ARI standard 885-90, Procedure for estimating occupied space sound levels in the application of air terminals and air outlets*. Arlington, Va: Air Conditioning and Refrigeration Institute.

ASHRAE. 1995. *1995 ASHRAE handbook—HVAC applications*, Chapter 43. Atlanta: American Society of Heating, Refrigerating and Air-Conditioning Engineers, Inc.

ASHRAE. 1991. *Algorithms for HVAC acoustics*. Atlanta: American Society of Heating, Refrigerating and Air-Conditioning Engineers, Inc.

Beranek, L.L. 1971. *Noise and vibration control*. New York: McGraw Hill.

Chapter 3
Noise Ratings and Acceptability Criteria

by *Warren Blazier*

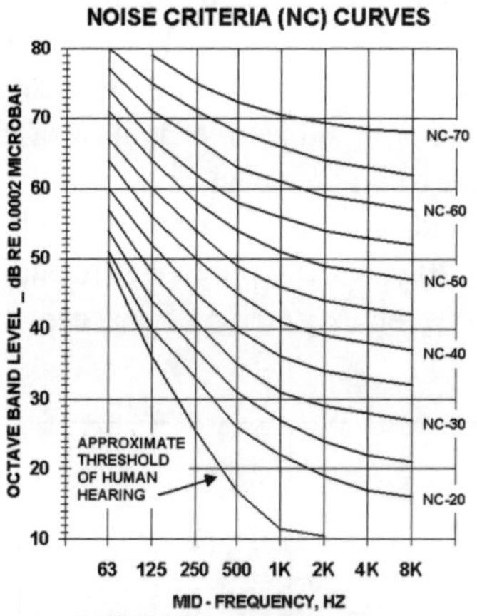

NC Criteria Curves

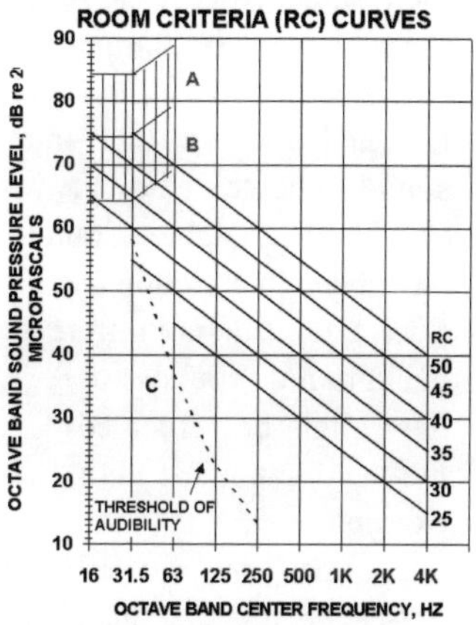

RC Criteria Curves

OVERVIEW

Several descriptors are presently used for the evaluation of noise from HVAC system operation. The ones most commonly used are:

- *A-weighted sound level, expressed in dB(A), such as 55 dB(A).* This rating is most frequently encountered in outdoor applications where compliance with community noise ordinances is a consideration. However, dB(A) is still occasionally used in specifying limits for indoor applications.
- *NC criteria, expressed as a rating number, such as NC-35.* NC criteria are most frequently used for rating HVAC noise in indoor applications where permissible noise limits have been specified on this basis.

- *RC criteria, expressed as a rating number plus a subjective quality descriptor, such as RC 35(N).* RC criteria are intended for use in indoor applications where the subjective quality of the sound, and not just the level at which it occurs, is to be taken into account.

Although tables of numerical criteria are available that list acceptable ratings in terms of one or more of the noise rating methods in common use (ASHRAE 1995; Harris 1991), such tables rarely explain the advantages or disadvantages of one descriptor over another for a given type of application. For example, if a recommended noise criterion has been met in a given application, it does not necessarily ensure that the occupant will find the environment satisfactory if the subjective character or quality of the noise is not addressed by the particular rating procedure used. Satisfaction can be a gamble if the specified noise criterion is only level-sensitive and does not take into account the subjective quality of the sound as perceived by the ear of the room occupant.

The A-weighted sound level and NC rating procedures, which have been in common use for over 30 years, are only level-sensitive. Such ratings do not differentiate between acceptable or unacceptable background sounds as they might be perceived by the human ear. For example, it is not uncommon for several noises having the same dB(A) or NC rating to rank significantly different when subjectively judged by a listener on a scale of relative acceptability. An example of the inability of either the dB(A) or NC rating methods to differentiate between acceptable and unacceptable sounds, on the basis of subjective quality, is illustrated in Figure 3-1.

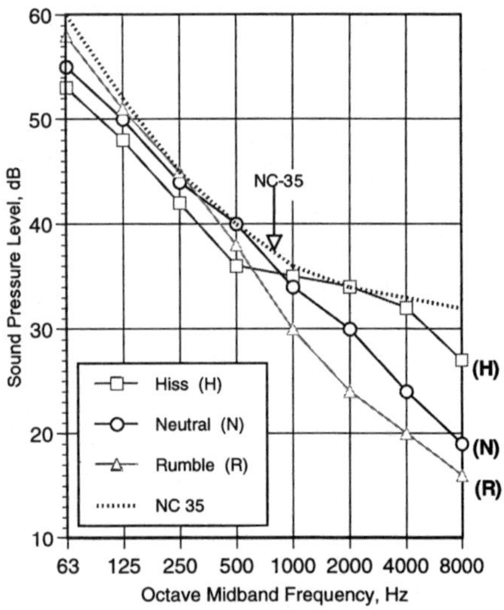

FIGURE 3-1 Three noise spectra having identical A-weighted sound levels (42 dB(A)) and identical NC ratings (NC 35).

In this example, three different noise spectra are shown that have identical A-weighted sound levels of 42 dB(A) and identical NC ratings of NC 35. However, the subjective character, or quality, of each noise spectrum illustrated is significantly different when perceived by the human ear. The spectrum labeled (H) sounds hissy, the spectrum labeled (R) sounds rumbly, while the spectrum labeled (N) is neutral in character, i.e., no one part of the spectrum dominates the character of the noise. These three spectra each receive a noise rating of NC 35 because the highest tangent NC curve in each instance is NC 35; the (H) spectrum is tangent at 2000 Hz, the (N) spectrum is tangent at 500 Hz, and the (R) spectrum is tangent at 250 Hz. (The NC rating, by convention, is determined by the highest NC curve tangent to the spectrum, independently of the frequency band in which it occurs.)

On the other hand, the RC noise rating procedure has the advantage of being not only level-sensitive, but also quality-sensitive. The RC rating procedure takes into account the subjective character of a noise such as "neutral," "rumble," or "hiss," by identifying these with the letter descriptors (N), (R), or (H), respectively, appended to the rating number. If the RC procedure had been used to rate the three spectra illustrated in Figure 3-1 above, the resulting ratings would have been RC-35(H) for the hissy-sounding spectrum, RC-35(N) for the neutral-sounding spectrum, and RC-31(R) for the rumbly sounding spectrum, thus identifying the differences in perceived sound quality among the three spectra.

The present industry trend is away from the use of either A-weighted sound levels or NC ratings. ASHRAE presently recommends only the use of the RC procedure for rating HVAC system noise in indoor spaces, especially if the application is sensitive to the quality of the sound.

Table 3-1 lists numerical RC(N) criteria, corresponding to various types of space occupancies, consistent with recommendations published in the *1995 ASHRAE Handbook—Applications*. The (N) designates a spectrum having a neutral, inoffensive sound quality. Details of the RC rating procedure and the guidelines that establish an (N) sound quality attribute are discussed in a subsequent section of this chapter.

Table 3-1
Design Guidelines for HVAC System Background Noise in Rooms

Room Types	RC(N) Criterion[a,b]
Residences, Apartments, Condominiums	25-35
Hotels/Motels	
Individual rooms or suites	25-35
Meeting/banquet rooms	25-35
Corridors, lobbies	35-45
Service/support areas	35-45
Office Buildings	
Executive and private offices	25-35
Conference rooms	25-35
Teleconference rooms	25 (max)
Open-plan offices	30-40
Corridors and lobbies	40-45
Hospitals and Clinics	
Private rooms	25-35
Wards	30-40
Operating rooms	25-35
Corridors and public areas	30-40
Performing Arts Spaces	
Drama theaters	25 (max)
Concert and recital halls[c]	
Music teaching studios	25 (max)
Music practice rooms	35 (max)
Laboratories (w/fume-hoods)	
Testing/research, minimal speech communication	45-55
Research, extensive telephone use, speech communication	40-50
Group teaching	35-45
Church, Mosque, Synagogue	
General assembly	25-35
With critical music programs[c]	

TABLE 3-1 (Continued)
Design Guidelines for HVAC System Background Noise in Rooms

Room Types	RC(N) Criterion[a,b]
Schools	
Classrooms up to 750 ft^2	40 (max)
Classrooms over 750 ft^2	35 (max)
Large lecture rooms, without speech amplification	35 (max)
Libraries	30-40
Courtrooms	
Unamplified speech	25-35
Amplified speech	30-40
Indoor Stadiums, Gymnasiums	
Gymnasiums and natatoriums[d]	40-50
Large seating-capacity spaces with speech amplification[d]	45-55

[a] The values and ranges are based on judgment and experience, not on quantitative evaluations of human reactions. They represent general limits of acceptability for typical building occupancies. Higher or lower values may be appropriate and should be based on a careful analysis of economics, space usage, and user needs.

[b] When the quality of sound in the space is important, specify criteria in terms of RC(N). If the quality of the sound in the space is of secondary concern, the criteria may be specified in terms of NC levels of similar magnitude.

[c] An experienced acoustical consultant should be retained for guidance on acoustically critical spaces (below RC 30) and for all performing arts spaces.

[d] RC or NC criteria for these spaces need only be selected for the desired speech and hearing conditions.

METHODS OF RATING HVAC SYSTEM NOISE

It is important to make a distinction between *source* noise ratings of individual components and *system* noise ratings of the combination of components when measured in the environment of the room occupant. In general, noise criteria are space-related and predicated upon achieving an acceptable room environment for a given type of occupancy. It is the system noise rating that must meet the noise criterion specified for a given type of space use.

On the other hand, the noise characteristics of system components are commonly expressed in terms of sound power level, which is not a space-related quantity. Therefore, component noise ratings cannot be directly compared to space-related criteria without first taking into account the noise reduction that occurs in the path between the source location in the system and the environment of the receiver, as discussed in Chapter 2.

A-Weighted Sound Level: Indoor Applications

The A-weighted sound level is a frequency-weighted sum of the energy contained in the sound pressure level spectrum expressed in decibel format. This weighting factor approximates the frequency response of the human ear at moderate sound levels, and, thus, tends to rank-order noises on the basis of comparative loudness as perceived by an average individual with normal hearing.

It is important to understand that "loudness" describes only the magnitude of a sound and that different noises may have the same A-weighted sound level or relative loudness but rank differently in the subjective opinion of a listener. This occurs because, in addition to loudness, the ear perceives differences in the frequency structure or "character" of sounds, which subjectively influences the comparative rank-ordering.

Returning to the example of three different spectra having the same A-weighted sound level illustrated previously in Figure 3-1, a typical listener would probably express a preference for the spectrum labeled (N) because its shape is usually inoffensive to the ear, if not too loud. However, either of the other spectrum shapes labeled (H) and (R) would likely be considered annoying due to the hissy character in one case and an excessive rumble in the other. Thus, a loudness-sensitive metric, such as the A-weighted sound level, cannot reliably rank-order noises on a subjective scale unless the frequency structure is nominally similar and the differences are mainly those of relative loudness. An example of this latter case is vehicular traffic noise, which is commonly rated in terms of A-weighted sound level.

Because HVAC system noises are widely variable with respect to frequency content and structure, the use of A-weighted sound level to specify criteria for indoor applications is not recommended except where dictated by present occupational health and safety noise exposure limits.

A-Weighted Sound Level: Outdoor Applications

Because of the present widespread use of A-weighted sound levels, dB(A), to specify outdoor environmental noise standards and regulations, the sound ratings of outdoor HVAC equipment, such as cooling towers, air-cooled condensing units, air-cooled chillers, etc., are frequently expressed in terms of A-weighted sound power level. However, such ratings must first be converted to A-weighted sound pressure level at some specified distance from the equipment before a comparison can be made with respect to specified environmental regulations. It is important to understand that simply meeting the property line noise limit prescribed by a regulation does not necessarily ensure that complaints in the neighborhood will be avoided, particularly if the quality of the noise is tonal in character or fluctuating in amplitude. These factors are not taken into account in the A-weighted rating.

NC, Noise Criteria Curves, NC-nn

The NC method of noise rating has been used extensively for over 30 years. The method is based on the use of a family of curves expressed in terms of octave-band sound pressure levels over the frequency range of 63 Hz to 8,000 Hz. Each curve in the family has a numerical designation, for example NC-40, which is keyed to a set of acceptability criteria expressed in terms of an identified space use. In conventional application by the industry, the NC rating is determined by plotting the octave-band spectrum of the noise in question on a family of NC curves and then assigning a numerical rating according to the highest NC curve that is just tangent to the spectrum. Although NC curves were originally defined in 5-NC increments, it has mistakenly become common practice to interpolate between the curves in 1-NC increments. *It is not a requirement of the rating procedure that the noise spectrum follow or approximate the actual shape of an NC curve. This is the principal reason that several noises that have the same NC rating may rank differently on the basis of subjective sound quality, as illustrated previously in Figure 3-1.*

In application to constant-volume HVAC systems, the past use of the NC rating procedure has proven to be relatively satisfactory for predicting or assessing the degree of potential occupant satisfaction. The primary reason is that a majority of the noise problems that occur in constant-volume systems are usually diffuser related and can be identified with excessive noise in the mid- to high-frequency range, thus controlling the magnitude of the NC rating. Problems with excessive noise in this frequency region can often be corrected, and the NC rating reduced to an acceptable value, by refining the system air-balance or by adding or re-sizing air diffusers.

With the introduction of the variable-air-volume (VAV) systems in the early 1980s, a new class of noise problems emerged that the NC rating procedure fails to detect. Most of these new problems typically result from excessive noise being produced in the frequency spectrum below 63 Hz, caused by a common practice of modulating air delivery by throttling at the fan and at air-control valves in the branch ductwork. The NC curves are not defined below the 63 Hz octave band, and for this reason they should not be used to rate noises that have a significant low-frequency content in the 16 Hz and 31.5 Hz octave bands.

Furthermore, an air diffuser selection in variable-volume systems tends to be made on the basis of the system operating at full air capacity. Thus, the diffuser noise levels at the reduced airflow requirements that occur during periods of normal occupancy (typically 50% to 80% of total capacity) may be as much as 15 dB lower than at full-volume design capacity. This reduction in mid- to high-frequency diffuser noise is often accompanied by a significant increase in low-frequency noise due to throttling at the fan and air-control terminals to match the changing demand. The overall result in the system as a whole is a low-frequency spectrum imbalance that, in many instances, the ear perceives as an offensive rumble.

Figure 3-2 illustrates an example of the typical result in a VAV system when the air volume demand is reduced to 65% of full capacity. The example assumes that an NC-35 noise criterion has been specified at full air capacity and that the system design meets this requirement.

The noise spectrum coded as the heavy solid line cor-

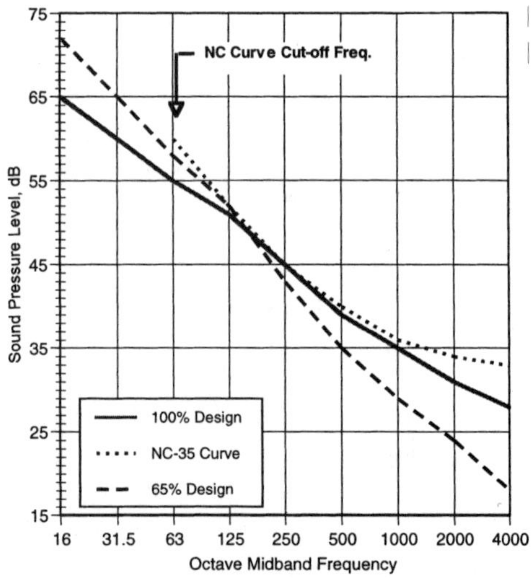

FIGURE 3-2 Effect of flow modulation on the spectrum shape and sound quality of HVAC noise in a variable-volume system.

responds to the full-volume flow condition. This is a relatively well-balanced neutral-sounding spectrum that meets the NC-35 design goal because of its tangency to the NC-35 criterion curve (dotted line) in the 250 Hz octave band.

The spectrum, shown as a heavy dashed line, illustrates changes in the shape of the noise spectrum that occurs when the airflow is reduced to 65% of full design capacity in a VAV system. Note that the level of low-frequency noise is increased due to throttling at the fan and air terminal devices, while at the same time the level of mid- to high-frequency noise is decreased because of the reduction in airflow through the diffusers. The combined result is a significantly unbalanced spectrum that is likely to be perceived as an annoying rumble because of the dominant low-frequency content. It is paradoxical that this spectrum also would be rated at NC-35 because of its tangency to the NC-35 curve at 125 Hz and the fact that the rating procedure ignores the level of the spectrum below 63 Hz. Thus, a room occupant frustrated by the rumbly quality of the sound environment at this "normal" operating condition might be difficult to convince that the system performance met the specified design goal.

Because the NC rating does not take spectrum shape into account or address the frequency range below 63 Hz, it is not recommended for the assessment of variable-volume HVAC systems if sound quality is an important consideration in the system design.

RC, Room Criteria Curves, RC-NN( )

The RC procedure for rating HVAC noise corrects several of the shortcomings of the A-weighted sound level and NC rating methods because the shape of the noise spectrum is taken into account in the assessment of sound quality. In addition, the frequency range of evaluation extends down to the 16 Hz octave band, thus addressing problems associated with excessive low-frequency noise.

The procedure for determining the RC rating of an octave-band noise spectrum provides valuable information for use in estimating the likely acceptability of a given system design. Four steps are required in the procedure:

1. The first step is to plot the spectrum to be rated and then calculate the arithmetic average of the octave-band levels in the 500 Hz, 1000 Hz, and 2000 Hz octave bands. This average value becomes the numerical part of the RC rat-

ing, which is important in addressing the speech communication or acoustical privacy requirements of the application that are affected by the sound pressure levels in this frequency region.

2. The second step is to plot a reference curve that has a slope of –5 dB/octave from 16 Hz to 4000 Hz, which passes through the 1000 Hz octave band at the average value determined in the first step. This reference curve represents the optimum shape of a "neutral-sounding" spectrum having the same degree of speech communication or acoustical privacy as the spectrum being rated.
3. The third step is to plot the limits above the reference curve, which cannot be exceeded by the noise spectrum being rated, in order to be classified as a neutral-sounding, subjectively inoffensive sound. The limits are +5 dB for the 16 Hz through 500 Hz octave bands and +3 dB for the 1000 Hz through 4000 Hz octave bands.
4. The final step is to note any deviations in the noise spectrum that exceed the level of the reference curve. If the deviations do not exceed 5 dB in the octave bands from 16 Hz to 500 Hz or 3 dB in the octave bands from 1000 Hz to 4000 Hz, the spectrum is classified as "neutral," and the letter descriptor (N) is appended to the numerical RC rating obtained in step one. However, if the deviations exceed 5 dB in the lower frequency range, the spectrum is classified as "rumbly" and assigned the letter descriptor (R). Conversely, if the deviations are in excess of 3 dB in the upper frequency range, the spectrum is classified as "hissy" and assigned the letter descriptor (H).[1]

An example using the RC rating procedure is illustrated in Figure 3-3. The spectrum to be rated is shown as the coded heavy solid line. The average of the sound pressure levels in the 500 Hz, 1000 Hz, and 2000 Hz octave bands is 35 dB, and this establishes the level of the –5 dB/octave reference curve in the 1000 Hz octave band (heavy dashed curve). The permissible low-frequency limit above the reference curve of +5 dB (16 Hz through 500 Hz) is plotted as the lighter dashed line; the permissible high-frequency limit above the reference curve (100 Hz through 4000 Hz) of +3 dB is

1. For a more complete description of the RC methodology and the RC Mark II updated version, see Chapters 43 and 52 of the *1995 and 1999 ASHRAE Handbook—Applications,* respectively.

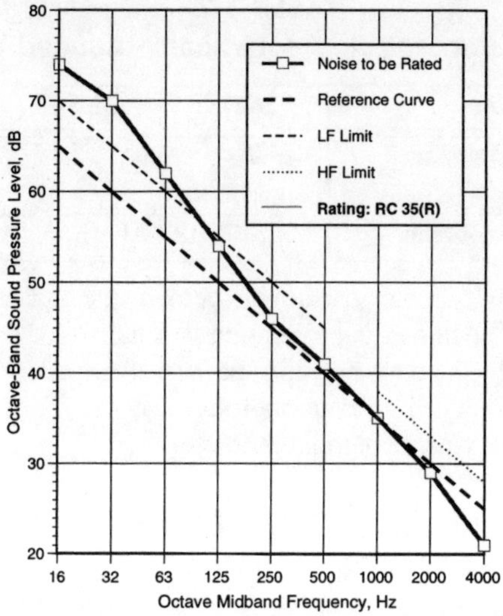

FIGURE 3-3 Example of steps to assign an RC rating to a noise spectrum. The spectrum shown above has a rating of RC 35(R). It has a rumbly character because the low-frequency limit curve is exceeded in the 16 Hz, 31.5 Hz, and 63 Hz octave bands.

plotted as the dotted line. This spectrum has a rating of RC 35(R), because the levels at 16 Hz, 31.5 Hz, and 63 Hz exceed the low-frequency limit curve.

With regard to achieving occupant satisfaction, it is obviously desirable to obtain an (N) rating in the assessment of sound quality. Should the spectrum receive an (R) or (H) rating, the potential for occupancy complaints exists. As a general rule, rumble and hiss complaints are likely if the levels of the spectrum exceed the reference curve by more than 5 dB or 3 dB, respectively.

CRITERIA FOR AVOIDING ACOUSTICALLY INDUCED LOW-FREQUENCY VIBRATION

The RC noise evaluation procedure also identifies sound pressure levels in the low-frequency region that are capable of producing acoustically-induced vibration in the walls and ceilings of rooms constructed of lightweight materials, such as wood or steel studs faced with gypsum-board. The octave-midband frequencies and corresponding sound pressure levels, where a problem due to acoustically-induced vibration is likely, are listed in Table 3-2. If the noise spectrum being rated has low-frequency sound pressure levels

TABLE 3-2
Criteria for Perceptible Acoustically-Induced Vibration

Criterion	16 Hz	31.5 Hz	63 Hz
Moderately Noticeable Vibrations	65 - 75 dB	65 - 75 dB	70 - 80 dB
Clearly Noticeable Vibrations	Above 75 dB	Above 75 dB	Above 80 dB

lying within the range shown below, the quality descriptor appended to the numerical RC rating is usually (RV). This indicates that the spectrum may not only be perceived as rumbly, but that acoustically-induced vibration of lightweight room surfaces and furnishings may be a potential problem.

EFFECT OF SMALL INCREMENTS IN NUMERICAL NOISE RATINGS

Although there may be a contractual requirement that a particular noise criterion or limit not be exceeded in a specified application, it should be recognized that people are not as precise as instruments in detecting differences in noise level. For example, the failure to achieve a specified criterion by 2 dB or 3 dB is normally inconsequential to a human observer, provided that the specified criterion or limit was appropriate to the application in the first place. However, exceeding specified criteria by 5 dB or more should be viewed as not conforming to the spirit of the noise specification.

As a general rule, when subjectively rank-ordering similar-sounding noises, an increase in level of about 5 dB is required to obtain reliable evidence that a significant subjective change has occurred. In other words, incremental differences of less than 5 dB in the level of a given noise are not generally sufficient for an average person to detect the change, particularly if the interval between comparisons is longer than a few seconds. However, if a prescribed noise criterion is missed by 5 dB or more, it is reasonable to assume that the "spirit" of the specification has not been met and occupant complaints are probable.

The relative significance of a 5 dB incremental change is reflected in nearly all of the criteria for noise assessment that have been developed over the years. For example, both the NC curves and the RC curves, as originally defined, were graduated in 5 dB increments. The same is true of most tables of acceptability criteria and application guidelines that have been published. Unfortunately, it has become common practice by the industry to interpolate in 1 dB increments between these criterion curves when rating room noise with respect to specified contractual requirements or in making comparisons among manufacturers' published acoustical data. Although this practice is at odds with the way people rank-order differences in noise level, it is nevertheless a fact of life that is not likely to change unless tolerances of at least 2 dB to 3 dB are incorporated in the specification of acoustical goals.

NOISE RATING OF COMPONENT NOISE SOURCES

As earlier discussed, there are presently no space-acceptability criteria for component noise ratings since the relative impact on the environment of the receiver depends entirely upon the source noise levels, their location in a system, and the noise attenuation that occurs along the path between source and receiver. Unfortunately, this places the manufacturers of HVAC components, such as air terminal and control devices, in a dilemma when asked to furnish ratings on the acoustical performance of their products. Most manufacturers can supply laboratory test data expressed in terms of sound power level (a measure of the acoustical energy emitted by the source and analogous to Btu/h in thermodynamics), but this is usually not what the typical user is requesting. The question really being asked is, "How much noise is your product going to contribute to the noise level in the environment served by my HVAC system?" Unfortunately, the answer depends upon how the system is laid out, what noise control measures are incorporated in the source to receiver path, and the acoustical characteristics of the receiving space. These are all factors over which a component manufacturer has no control.[2]

FIELD MEASUREMENT OF ROOM SOUND PRESSURE LEVEL

In the commissioning of HVAC systems in buildings, it is frequently required that the achievement of a specified room noise criterion be demonstrated. Measurement procedures are often not specified for obtaining the data necessary to demonstrate this qualification. This leads to considerable confusion when the various

2. Industry associations, such as ARI, are presently trying to develop methods of converting component noise ratings, expressed in terms of sound power level, to space-related noise criteria by defining default values for noise reduction in system applications for various configurations of equipment. For specific details, refer to the discussion of individual system components in other chapters of this book.

interested parties each make measurements using different methodologies. The results often do not agree. The problem is that most real rooms encountered in typical field situations exhibit some point-to-point variation in sound pressure level. Thus, measurements made at different locations in a room will not usually be the same.

Except where there are audible tonal components in the noise, the differences in the measured sound pressure level at several locations in a room are not usually large enough to be significant to the casual observer (±2 dB). However, when audible tonal components are present, the variations due to standing waves may exceed 5 dB, and these are generally noticeable to the average listener, depending upon their location in the room.

Unfortunately, in the commissioning process, where precise limits usually are established as the basis for demonstrating compliance, the outcome can be controversial unless the measurement procedure to be followed has been specified in detail. At the present time, there is no general agreement within the industry regarding an acoustical measurement procedure for commissioning HVAC systems. However, ARI has taken an initial step in this direction by incorporating a "suggested procedure for field verification of NC/RC levels" in *ARI Standard 885-90, Procedure for Estimating Occupied Space Sound Levels in the Application of Air Terminals and Air Outlets*.

ARI Standard 885-90 recommends defining the octave-band room sound pressure level of the spectrum as the energy average of each octave-band level measured at four specified points in the space of concern. The recommended locations of these four points are illustrated in Figure 3-4.

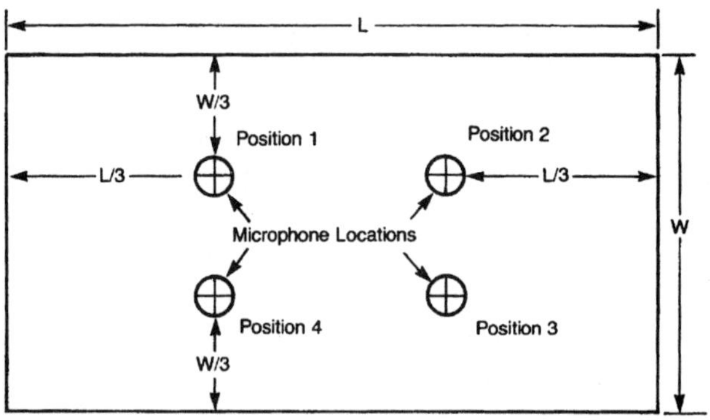

FIGURE 3-4 Recommended microphone locations for measuring the average room sound pressure level. Each microphone location is 5 ft above the floor.

ARI Standard 885-90 also provides a procedure for processing the data obtained at each measurement location to calculate the energy-averaged level in each octave band over the frequency range of interest. Thus, the average octave-band spectrum of the noise can be determined for comparison to a specified room noise criterion.

Those directly involved in the specification and commissioning process are encouraged to use ARI 885-90 procedures for most HVAC applications to avoid commissioning controversies.

REFERENCES

ASHRAE. 1995. *1995 ASHRAE handbook—HVAC Applications*, Chapter 43, Table 2. Atlanta: American Society of Heating, Refrigerating and Air-Conditioning Engineers, Inc.

Harris, C.M. 1991. Handbook of acoustical measurements and noise control, 3d ed., Table 43.1. New York: McGraw-Hill.

Chapter 4
Fan Noise Characteristics Tutorial

by *Warren Blazier*

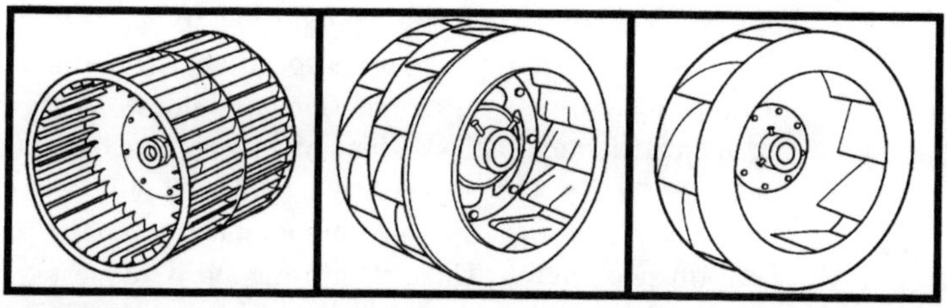

OVERVIEW

This chapter describes both the aerodynamic performance and acoustical characteristics of the fan types normally used in HVAC systems. The fans included in this discussion are the forward-curved, backward-inclined flat or airfoil blade, plenum (plug), vaneaxial, and propeller types.

VARIABILITY AND RELIABILITY OF AVAILABLE FAN SOUND POWER DATA

The sources of acoustical data provided by most manufacturers of fan equipment usually can be classified in one of the three following categories:

1. **Calculated data, using generalized equations published in most editions of the *ASHRAE Handboo*k prior to 1995.** ASHRAE no longer recommends using this methodology as a basis for the noise control design of HVAC systems because the level of uncertainty is simply too great, particularly in application to the design of variable-air-vol-

ume (VAV) systems. Furthermore, it was mistakenly assumed in the development of these generalized equations that the level and shape of both the inlet and discharge noise spectra were similar and that each was 3 dB less than the calculated total octave-band sound power levels. This is an oversimplification, and their true relationship to each other can only be validated by measuring each side separately.

2. **Calculated data based on extrapolations permitted by *AMCA Standard 301-90, Methods for Calculating Fan Sound Ratings from Laboratory Test Data.*** These calculations are based on test data obtained from a fan of a given size when measured in accordance with *AMCA Standard 300-85, Reverberant Room Method for Sound Testing of Fans*. A conversion procedure is specified that permits the data obtained on the tested fan to be used in estimating the acoustical characteristics of fans of a larger size but within the same family. The conversion is permitted only between two fans operating at the same point on their respective air performance curves. Thus, if information is requested on an untested fan, with respect to operation at several points on its characteristic air performance curve, measured data must be available on the tested reference fan at similar operating points in order for the calculations to be valid.

   The reliability of the data generated using this conversion methodology is considered by AMCA to be better than that obtained using the generalized ASHRAE equations discussed above. However, it must be emphasized that the reliability of the data submitted by a fan manufacturer depends upon how closely the procedures of AMCA Standard 301-90 were adhered to in developing the submittal. If the distribution of data points along the performance curve of the tested fan were too sparse, the reliability of the conversions to fans of a larger size could be highly questionable.

   The data submitted by most fan manufacturers usually will be based on AMCA Standard 301-90 because it is unlikely that the available measured database will be extensive enough to cover all fan sizes at a variety of operating points. However, in acoustically critical applications, it is not uncommon for the engineer to require that the data submitted for approval be obtained from tests on the actual fan size that is to be used, when operating at the specified point on the characteristic fan curve, as described below.

3. **Measured data obtained from specific laboratory tests of the specified fan at a specified operating point.** Applicable procedures are *AMCA Standard 300-85, Reverberant Room Method for Sound Testing of Fans* or *AMCA Standard 330-86, Laboratory Method of Testing In-Duct Sound Power Measurement Procedure for Fans.* In principle, laboratory tests on the specified fan are far more reliable than those extrapolated from tests on a fan of a different size using AMCA Standard 301-90.
   However, it must be cautioned that several of the standard setups for sound testing per AMCA 300 are for the determination of the total sound power output of the fan. This is a meaningless test for most field applications because, in order to incorporate appropriate noise control measures in the system design, it is essential to have data pertaining to both inlet and discharge noise separately. The level and spectrum shape of inlet vs. discharge noise can be significantly different; these are not equal and simply 3 dB less than the total, as incorrectly assumed in some manufacturers' literature.

FAN AS A STAND-ALONE SYSTEM COMPONENT

When a fan is installed as a separate component in a built-up HVAC system, rather than as part of an air-handling package, its performance may closely approximate the manufacturer's submittal data, provided that the inlet and discharge conditions at the fan are aerodynamically optimized. These are the conditions under which the fan would have been tested per AMCA Standard 300-85. However, the test results cannot be expected to be duplicated in the field if the inlet and discharge conditions are badly configured. Whenever a fan is to be installed as a component of a built-up system, the engineer may have the option of negotiating sufficient space allowance to permit the design of proper inlet and discharge duct transitions, and thus avoid undesirable system effects that may degrade the fan performance both aerodynamically and acoustically. This option typically is not available when the fan is part of a packaged HVAC unit because of space limitations influenced by competitive marketing pressures.

FAN AS A COMPONENT OF PACKAGED AIR-HANDLING EQUIPMENT

A fan incorporated in packaged air-handling equipment usually does not perform as efficiently as when tested as a stand-alone component in accordance with *AMCA Standard 210-85, Laboratory Methods of Testing Fans for Rating,* for air performance and AMCA Standard 300-85 for acoustics. The reason is that the packaged inlet and discharge geometry rarely duplicates the idealized conditions of the laboratory setup. Thus, because of the degraded airflow, the fan efficiency is typically reduced and the noise of operation increased by 5 dB to 10 dB in the frequency range below about 250 Hz.

In the design of packaged air-handling equipment, with strong emphasis typically placed on compactness, it is usually not possible to optimize the fan entrance and exit geometry. As a result, the actual fan performance, both aerodynamically and acoustically, usually will not agree with the AMCA-300 data submitted by the manufacturer of the fan. Instead, the specification of Draft ARI Standard 260P, Sound Rating of Air Moving and Conditioning Equipment, is recommended when requesting data on the acoustical performance of packaged air-handling equipment. Although this standard utilizes test procedures similar to AMCA 300-85, measurements of the inlet, discharge, and radiated noise of the package are determined as separate components of the total noise produced by the package.

APPLYING MANUFACTURERS' DATA TO BUILDING SYSTEM DESIGN

As with any laboratory test procedure, there are always measurement uncertainties to be taken into account when reporting data. Also, uncertainty in low-frequency acoustical data using measurement procedures, such as those specified by AMCA 300-85 and by Draft ARI 260P, is very sensitive to the physical size of the test chamber. The larger the test chamber is, the less the uncertainty is in the measurements. As a general rule, Table 4-1 illustrates the potential magnitude of uncertainties that should be taken into account when applying manufacturers' fan test data to an HVAC system design.

TABLE 4-1
Expected Uncertainties in Fan Noise Data

Octave-Midband Frequency (Hz)	Measurement Uncertainty
Below 63	± 8 dB
63	± 5 dB
125	± 3 dB
250	± 3 dB
Above 250	± 3 dB

MANUFACTURERS' SOUND RATING PROCEDURES AND PRACTICES

OCTAVE-BAND SOUND POWER LEVEL, dB WITH RESPECT TO 10^{-12} WATT

The customary format of the data provided by most manufacturers of centrifugal and vaneaxial fan equipment, and some manufacturers of propeller fan equipment, is usually expressed in terms of octave-band sound power level (L_w) with respect to 10^{-12} watt, over a frequency range of 8 octave bands, extending from 63 Hz to 8000 Hz. One-third octave-band data is also available from some manufacturers, if requested. One-third octave-band readings have the advantage of permitting the identification of tonal components in the noise spectrum so that appropriate precautions can be taken in the system noise control design. Vaneaxial fan equipment typically produces at least one, and often two or more, of these subjectively annoying tonal components. Thus, it is always advisable to request one-third octave-band data when considering an application that uses vaneaxial fans.

RELATIVE LOUDNESS IN SONES VS. ANNOYANCE

Sones

The sone is a unit of subjective loudness. It is a linear measure of the relative loudness of a signal with respect to a 1000 Hz reference tone at a level of 40 dB, which by definition has a loudness of one sone. In principle, a magnitude of two sones is twice as loud as one sone; four sones are four times as loud as one sone, but only twice as loud as two sones, etc.

Unfortunately, outside the laboratory the sone has little practical application. One reason is that there is no universal agreement on the appropriate procedure to use in calculating sone ratings. There are two significantly different procedures in use at the present time (ISO 1975), each of which provides a different numerical result! Although the sone ratios tend to be similar when using either of these procedures to compare the relative loudness of one sound with respect to another, the sone values of the individual sounds may significantly differ between the two methods. Therefore, one should not compare sone ratings unless it is known that the same calculation procedure was used.

Furthermore, a noise rating expressed in sones is of little value in engineering a noise-control solution to a problem because the spectral distribution of the signal is an unknown. Unfortunately, some manufacturers of power roof ventilation equipment have departed from the convention adopted by the remainder of the fan industry and have chosen to rate the noise level of this equipment in sones rather than in terms of octave-band sound power levels. This optional method of rating is nevertheless permitted by *AMCA Standard 301-90, Methods for Calculating Fan Sound Ratings from Laboratory Test Data.*

However, because AMCA Standard 301-90 specifies a procedure for the sone calculation, which first requires determining the *octave-band sound power level spectrum* of the noise source, the octave-band information is available and should be requested to facilitate the design of appropriate noise control measures for the HVAC system application.

Annoyance

Except, perhaps, within the scientific community, most people mistakenly tend not to differentiate between the terms "loudness" and "annoyance" and assume that both mean essentially the same. This is not true. For example, it is quite possible for two different fan designs to have identical sone ratings (loudness) but to be assigned dramatically different rankings on a scale of subjective annoyance. The reason is that the two fans may have significantly different spectral distributions of sound pressure level. The fan that is less annoying may have a broad-band distribution of sound energy that is not perceived by the listener as offensive. Conversely, the more annoying fan likely has a spectrum where more of the energy is concentrated at a single frequency, and this may be perceived by the listener as a very annoying tonal component. Most bathroom exhaust fans are an example of this latter category.

TYPES OF FANS USED IN HVAC SYSTEMS

In many ducted applications of HVAC equipment, typical operating requirements usually permit a choice among five generic fan types: forward-curved, backward-inclined flat or airfoil blade, plenum ("plug"), and vaneaxial. The use of propeller fan equipment is typically limited to nonducted applications where the fan operates near "free" air delivery.

There are, of course, many considerations that influence the particular type of fan chosen for a given application. When operating, noise level is an important consideration and two factors are of primary concern. The first is the fan efficiency at the system operating point; in general, the higher the fan efficiency, the lower the noise level in the application. Second, the frequency content and characteristic shape of the noise spectrum associated with a particular fan type is of concern because this strongly influences the frequency range where noise control measures are required to achieve an acceptably quiet system.

NOISE CHARACTERISTICS OF FORWARD-CURVED CENTRIFUGAL FANS

Forward-curved fans are best suited to application in low static-pressure HVAC systems (up to two inches of water). They are occasionally employed in medium static-pressure systems (about two to four inches of water), particularly where considerations of lower first cost and smaller physical size take precedence over both operating efficiency and noise level. The peak efficiency that can be achieved by a fan of forward-curved design is the lowest among all fan types that might be considered for similar applications.

VARIABILITY WITH POINT OF OPERATION ON THE FAN AIR PERFORMANCE CURVE

The typical shape of the air performance curve of a forward-curved fan is illustrated in Figure 4-1. The level and character of the noise of operation depends upon the point at which the system resistance curve intersects the fan air performance curve. The quietest point of operation is in the region of peak fan efficiency, corresponding to an intersection with the system resistance curve labeled (a).

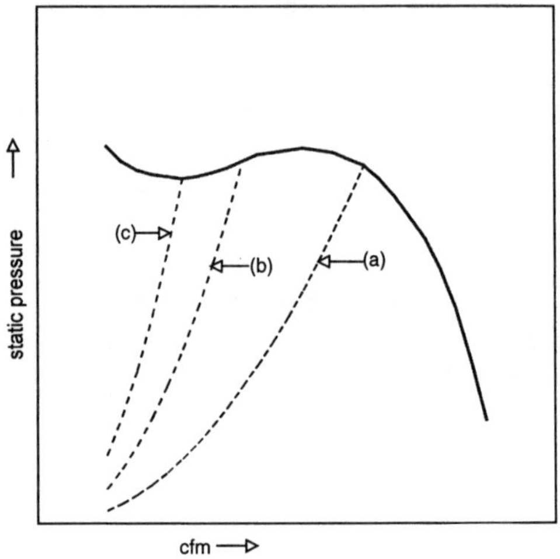

FIGURE 4-1 Air performance curve of a typical forward-curved fan. The system resistance curve, (a), intersects the fan curve in the region of peak efficiency, which is the quietest point of operation. The system resistance curve, (b), intersects the fan curve in the region of "rotating stall," causing rumble. The system resistance curve, (c), intersects the fan curve in the "surge" region, causing low-frequency fluctuating noise.

The system resistance curve labeled (b) intersects the fan curve in the region of "rotating stall" and causes a substantial increase in the level of low-frequency rumble and a tonal component at about two-thirds the fan rpm/60 Hz. An intersection with the system resistance curve labeled (c) corresponds to the "surge" region of the fan performance, which not only contributes to a substantial increase in the level of low-frequency noise but also typically possesses an annoying amplitude-modulated, fluctuating time pattern that is perceived as rumble.

Operation to the right of peak efficiency (farther out on the fan curve) also causes a general increase in the level of fan noise, with the largest changes occurring in the mid- and high-frequency range (hiss) and at the blade-passage frequency (number of fan blades × rpm/60).

AMCA Standard 300-85 does not require measurements to be made below the 63 Hz octave band. Thus, the acoustical data provided by most fan manufacturers generally will not disclose the presence of potential low-frequency noise problems in the 16 Hz and 31.5 Hz octave bands.

Fan aerodynamic instability caused by operation in the region of stall or surge (regions (b) to (c) of the fan curve) can be identified acoustically with a marked increase in the level of low-frequency noise in the 16 Hz and 31.5 Hz octave bands. However, it is not customary for manufacturers to test in the stall or surge region of the fan curve because this is definitely not a recommended range of operation in the normal course of fan selection. Problems in the field with fan stall or surge are usually due to the selection of an oversized fan or caused by abnormal pressure losses introduced by poor entrance and exit conditions in the external ductwork, often called *system-effects*.

Constant Volume vs. Variable Volume Applications

Forward-curved fans are best suited for application in constant-volume systems, where the system resistance is constant and an appropriate selection of fan size can be made to ensure that the operating point lies within the most efficient and acoustically favorable region of the fan curve (near the peak efficiency point). However, when used in variable-volume applications, forward-curved fans have a high risk of operating in an unstable region of the fan curve as the system resistance is changed and the airflow is choked-down to meet the demand. The level of risk depends upon the magnitude of flow reduction requirements and the method used to achieve it. The highest risk occurs when variable inlet vanes or discharge dampers are employed; the least risk is encountered when using variable-speed control.

Variable-Volume System Applications

Variable Inlet Vanes (VIV)

The aerodynamic performance of forward-curved fans, and hence the operating noise level, is extremely sensitive to the fan inlet geometry. The lowest noise level and the highest aerodynamic efficiency are achieved when the inlet flow is symmetrical and allowed to enter the fan naturally without obstruction. Whenever variable inlet vanes are added to the fan for flow modulation, the shape of the fan performance curve is altered, the operating efficiency of the fan is reduced, and the fan may become 5 dB to 10 dB noisier in the low-frequency range.

Even when the inlet vanes are in the full-open position, the disturbance produced in the inlet flow profile typically increases the operating sound level of the fan by about 5 dB on average. As the vanes close down to reduce air delivery, the distortion in the shape of the characteristic fan curve has the effect of shifting the operating point in the direction of rotating stall or surge and increasing the level of low-frequency noise. At some point in the vane closure cycle, the fan may become unstable and may be accompanied by a substantial increase in the level of low-frequency noise concentrated in the 16 Hz and 31.5 Hz octave bands.

In some VIV applications, the unstable region of fan operation is encountered before the reduced airflow requirements are satisfied. Packaged rooftop equipment is particularly susceptible to a problem of this nature because of the widespread use of double-inlet, double-width forward-curved fans fitted with variable inlet vanes for flow modulation. It is not uncommon for the required airflow, in order to maintain comfort during normal occupancy periods, to be significantly lower than the maximum fan capacity that is generally used as the basis for design and fan selection. Thus, the inlet vanes are most often only partially open, increasing the possibility for the fan to enter a stall or surge mode of operation.

Variable-Speed Drive (VSD)

Significantly lower levels of noise can be achieved if the flow modulation is accomplished by reducing the fan speed rather than by operating at constant speed and throttling with variable inlet vanes. There is also another advantage to VSD, as opposed to VIV control. The fan selection can be made such that the operating point remains at or near the point of peak efficiency over the entire range of flow modulation. Table 4-2 illustrates the potential noise reduction achieved by reducing fan speed.[1]

TABLE 4-2
Noise Reduction by Reducing Fan Speed

Fan Speed Ratio	Noise Reduction, dB
1.0	0
0.8	5
0.6	11
0.4	20
0.2	35

1. Fan noise tends to vary approximately as [10 × log (cfm)] + [20 × log (p)] over most of the frequency range. Since cfm varies directly with speed and p varies with the square of the speed, this is equivalent to [50 × log (speed)].

Because the shape of the fan characteristic curve changes little as airflow is reduced by reducing speed, it is possible to modulate over a much greater flow range without encountering flow instability. Furthermore, because the geometry of the inlet flow to the fan is undisturbed by the presence of throttling vanes, the usual 5 dB penalty of a VIV-obstructed inlet need not be applied.

However, even with a variable-speed drive, there is usually a limit on the magnitude of airflow reduction possible before the fan undergoes rotating stall or surge. This is due to the distortion in the shape of the system resistance curve caused by the static-pressure controller. The problem can be avoided in many cases by not setting the static-pressure controller at a value higher than absolutely necessary to meet the system requirements.

NOISE CHARACTERISTICS OF BACKWARD-INCLINED, FLAT- OR AIRFOIL-BLADE FANS

The backward-inclined flat-blade (BI) and airfoil-blade (AF) fan designs have similar air performance characteristics suitable for application in medium and high static-pressure HVAC systems (about three to six inches of water). The airfoil-blade fan design has the highest aerodynamic efficiency and potentially lowest operating noise level in comparison to other generic fan types that might be considered for the same application. The normal shape of the aerodynamic performance characteristic of a BI/AF fan is a smooth curve without the pronounced "knee" that is typical of forward-curved or vaneaxial designs. It is less vulnerable to the onset of instability problems when operating somewhat to the left of the peak-efficiency point. Thus, the BI/AF fans are perhaps the most forgiving of the other fan types with respect to the ability to operate over a broader range of the air performance curve without becoming unstable or producing excessive noise.

VARIABILITY WITH POINT OF OPERATION ON THE FAN AIR PERFORMANCE CURVE

The characteristic shape of the typical air performance curve of BI and AF fans is illustrated in Figure 4-2. The quietest point of operation on the fan curve is in the region of peak efficiency, near the intersection of system resistance curve (a) with the fan characteristic curve. Operation to the right of peak efficiency, farther out on the fan curve in the direction of the system resistance curve (b),

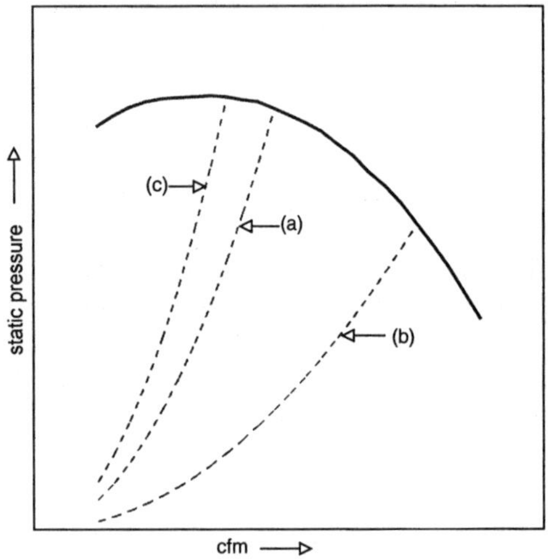

FIGURE 4-2 Typical air performance curve of backward-inclined flat-blade or airfoil-blade fans. System resistance curve (a) intersects the fan curve in the region of peak efficiency. The normal range of fan selection is between curves (a) and (b). A surge condition typically develops when operated in the region to the left of curve (c).

results in a moderate increase in mid- and high-frequency noise levels above about 250 Hz.

Thus, many engineers tend to make a selection in the direction of a somewhat undersized fan to avoid problems with surge in case the effective system resistance turns out to be significantly higher than anticipated. This reasoning also has acoustical advantages because it is much easier to deal with the increased mid- and high-frequency noise of an undersized fan operating at some distance out on the air performance curve than it is to cope with the low-frequency problems introduced by an oversized fan operating too far back on the air performance curve. However, operating too far left of the peak efficiency point, on the flat portion of the air performance curve near the intersection with system curve (c), will result in a type of flow instability termed "surge."[2] In a surge operating

2. The distinction between rotating stall (breakdown and partial reversal of flow inside a part of the fan wheel) and a surge condition (time modulation of the mean flow in the airway path) typically can be diagnosed in the field by measuring the static pressure rise across the fan. If the static pressure is relatively constant but there is an abnormal amount of vibration likely, the fan is in rotating stall. If the pressure rise across the fan exhibits large fluctuations in magnitude with time, a surge condition is indicated.

mode, large fluctuations in air delivery occur that tend to be pulsed or time-modulated at a rate dependent upon the dynamic response of the external system to changes in air volume. The fluctuation rate can vary from about one per second (short distribution system) to one in which the period per cycle approaches 30 or more seconds (extended distribution system with multiple branches). Considerable vibration also accompanies fan operation in a surge mode. Acoustically, a surge condition is identified by a substantial increase in low-frequency noise levels below 100 Hz that undergo large fluctuations in amplitude as a function of time (rumble).

A surge condition in a BI/AF fan is usually only encountered if the fan is either oversized for the application, operating at a substantially reduced flow rate under the control of variable inlet vanes, or provoked by unanticipated external system effects that significantly increase the effective system resistance.

Acoustical and Energy-Conservation Considerations in Application to Variable-volume Systems

Two control options are typically available for flow-modulation of BI/AF fans in variable-volume systems. These are the use of variable inlet vanes at constant fan speed and variable-speed control of a fixed fan geometry. Of the two options, variable-speed drive is by far a better engineering choice because both the operating noise level and the power consumed by the fan are significantly lower at comparable reduced-flow conditions.

Variable Inlet Vanes (VIV)

In most applications of BI/AF fans in variable-volume systems, the selection of fan size is usually based on peak-load design air capacity. However, peak load conditions occur only during a small fraction of the system operating time, and the requirements to maintain comfort during periods of normal occupancy usually lie within the range of 50% to 80% of peak design capacity. When variable inlet vanes are used to modulate air volume, such as to the midpoint of normal occupancy requirements (about 65% of peak capacity), the fan consumes about 88% of the horsepower required to deliver the peak air capacity. The fan noise level at this reduced flow condition is usually similar to that at peak design capacity or somewhat higher because of the reduction in fan efficiency caused by the throttling action of the inlet vanes. Furthermore, because the vanes obstruct the fan inlet, even in the wide-open position, the fan sound level at a given flow volume is typically about 5 dB higher than that of a similar fan operating at the same speed but installed without inlet vanes.

It is important to recognize that the range over which the fan air volume can be safely modulated using variable inlet vanes is limited. Usually, if the vanes are closed down beyond a certain point, the fan can shift into a surge operating mode that is accompanied by a dramatic increase in the level of low-frequency noise below 100 Hz. Most manufacturers provide performance curves for fans fitted with inlet vanes that indicate the region in which the fan is likely to be unstable and operate in a surge mode, as a function of vane setting. However, it must be understood that the manufacturer's information is normally based on tests made with ideal fan entrance and exit conditions and that these are often not duplicated in typical field applications of fan equipment. Consequently, the stable operating range of flow modulation in a field situation is likely to be less than indicated by the fan curves furnished by the manufacturer.

Whenever a BI or AF fan operates in the unstable region of its air performance curve, the low-frequency noise level (rumble) can increase by as much as 10 dB to 15 dB in the 16 Hz and 31.5 Hz octave bands. In addition, the fan vibration level may become excessive. Unfortunately, the excessive level of vibration due to a surging fan is often misinterpreted as resulting from an abnormal amount of mechanical imbalance in the rotating system. Field examples are frequently reported where a high level of fan vibration, initially attributed to a mechanical unbalance, was not corrected by measures taken to rebalance the fan equipment. Ultimately, the problem was traced to fan surge, caused either by the system operating too far to the left of the peak efficiency point, or because of an oversized fan that required an excessive degree of vane closure to achieve the reduced airflow requirement.

Variable-Speed Drive

By selecting the variable-speed drive option to modulate airflow, the horsepower required to operate the system at 65% of peak air volume is only about 27% of the requirement to deliver the full design air quantity. The fan sound level at 65% of total air volume is also approximately 9 dB lower than that at the operating speed corresponding to total design air delivery. Furthermore, because there are no variable inlet vanes to distort the entering flow profile, the fan sound level is also about an additional 5 dB less than if inlet

TABLE 4-3
Comparison of Changes in Fan Sound Level and Shaft Horsepower to Operate System at 65% of Design Flow Volume*

Flow Control Option	Change in Sound Level *re* Design Air Volume of Fan w/o VIV Assembly	Change in Horsepower *re* Design Air Volume of Fan w/o VIV Assembly
100% Volume Without Variable Inlet Vanes	"X"	"Y"
65% Volume Using Variable Inlet Vanes (VIV)	"X" + 5 dBA	88% "Y"
65% Volume Using Variable Speed Drive (VSD)	"X" – 9 dBA	27% "Y"

* Note: Comparison is relative to the sound level, "X," and shaft horsepower, "Y," at 100% flow volume for a fan without a variable inlet vane assembly installed.

vanes were present but operated in the full-open position. Thus, the level of fan noise, when supplying 65% of total air capacity, is about 14 dB less with variable speed control than if the same operating condition were achieved using variable inlet vanes. Clearly, there is a dramatic acoustical advantage to using a variable-speed drive to modulate air capacity. Also, the reduction in power consumption to operate the system is substantial. A comparison between the two methods of flow modulation at 65% of design capacity is shown in Table 4-3.

When using fan speed to modulate airflow in a typical VAV system, the intersection of the system curve with a point on the fan curve will shift slightly to the left as airflow is reduced, but the characteristic shape of the fan curve is not altered. This shift in the intersection of the system curve with the fan curve occurs because the normal "square-law" shape of the system curve is distorted by the action of the static-pressure controller. Because of this, it is possible to cause the fan to surge at drastically reduced airflows. However, if the selection of fan size is appropriate to the application, a surge condition is rarely encountered over the range of flow modulation normally required.

NOISE CHARACTERISTICS OF PLENUM (PLUG) FANS

The plenum, or "plug" fan, is an application of a single-inlet BI or AF fan impeller housed in a sound absorptive plenum rather than in the customary volute scroll. Plenum fans are rapidly gaining popularity for use in packaged air-handling equipment because of the space-saving feature offered by eliminating the need for an extended duct transition between the discharge side of the fan and the connection to the air distribution system. The fan efficiency obtainable with a plenum fan is usually less than that of the generic BI/AF fan installed in a volute housing. However, some manufacturers claim that the operating efficiency of a plenum fan can approach that which is achievable with a volute-housed fan by using a modified airfoil impeller with a specially designed inlet bell to ensure that a uniform entering air profile is present at the fan inlet. The shape of the characteristic air performance curve of a plenum fan is similar in most respects to that illustrated in Figure 4-2 for the generic BI/AF fan.

A plenum fan uses a single-inlet impeller assembly that is mounted inside a plenum enclosure. The inlet to the fan is a bell-mouthed assembly mounted flush to one sidewall of the plenum. The fan pressurizes the plenum, and discharge air is obtained from one or more taps in the other sidewalls. The plenum fan design is applicable to all HVAC systems that might otherwise use a generic, scroll-housed BI/AF fan. In draw-through applications, the fan discharge is ducted to the system by a connection to the top or sidewall of the discharge plenum. In blow-through applications, the discharge plenum is extended to incorporate the heating/cooling coils, and a connection to the external system is made by tapping the plenum top or sidewall on the downstream side of the coils. There are significant acoustical advantages to using a blow-through as opposed to a draw-through configuration.

Variability with Point of Operation on Fan Air Performance Curve

The acoustical characteristics of a plenum fan are sensitive to the point of operation on the fan curve in a manner generally similar to the BI and AF fans described above. The quietest point of operation on the fan curve is in the region of peak efficiency. Operation to the right of peak efficiency (farther out on the fan curve) results in a moderate increase in the level of mid- and high-frequency noise, whereas operation too far to the left of peak efficiency can create a surge condition. The acoustical advantages of a plenum fan, in comparison to volute-housed BI and AF fans, stem from the fact that the sound absorptive treatment incorporated in the discharge plenum results in significantly lower levels of discharge noise being coupled to the external system. However, with respect to the magnitude of inlet noise, there is no difference between a plenum fan and a volute-housed BI/AF fan.

With respect to flow modulation using either variable inlet vanes or a variable-speed drive, the plenum fan behaves no differently than the volute-housed BI and AF fans discussed above. However, in addition to these two methods of flow modulation, a third option exists because of the use of a single-inlet impeller. Although this option is known by several proprietary names, in principle it is a controllable device centered about the axis of fan rotation, which moves between the back-plate of the fan impeller and the inlet to alter the effective width of the impeller. In comparison to variable inlet vanes, it is, acoustically, a more desirable method of flow modulation, but it does not achieve the operating efficiency and lower noise levels resulting from the use of a variable-speed drive.

Fan Inlet

The inlet geometry of a plenum fan is in most respects identical to that of a BI/AF fan housed in a volute scroll. Therefore, the acoustical characteristics at the fan inlet are similar to those of the generic BI/AF fan.

Fan Discharge

The noise spectrum occurring at the discharge connection to a plenum fan contains significantly less mid- and high-frequency energy than is present on the discharge side of a volute-housed BI/AF fan. This is because the sidewalls of the plenum are usually faced with acoustical material that is an efficient absorber of mid- and high-frequency noise. In addition, there can also be significant low-frequency sound attenuation, depending upon the size and configuration of the discharge plenum. It is not unusual to achieve a low-frequency noise reduction on the order of 10 dB with an appropriately sized discharge plenum.

NOISE CHARACTERISTICS OF VANEAXIAL FANS

Vaneaxial fans are suitable for application in low, medium, and high static-pressure HVAC systems. They have a particular advantage where the requirements are for straight-through flow in a compact installation. The aerodynamic efficiency achievable by a vaneaxial fan, installed with optimum entering and exit conditions, is among the highest of the generic fan types typically used in HVAC systems. Vaneaxial fans characteristically produce the least low-frequency noise of any of the fan types; for that reason, they are often used in applications where the greater noise level produced at high frequencies can be managed with passive or active sound attenuation devices. Vaneaxial fans are the most sensitive to inlet flow obstructions, such as inlet guide vanes for flow modulation or external platform-mounted motor drives. Such inlet obstructions cause a substantial increase in noise at the blade-pass frequency.

Variability with Point of Operation on Fan Air Performance Curve

The mid-frequency noise spectrum of a vaneaxial fan usually contains a pronounced peak at the *blade-passage frequency.* The blade-passage frequency is the product of the number of fan blades times the fan rpm/60. For example, a fan having 12 blades and operating at 1800 rpm produces a blade-passage frequency at 360 Hz.

When nonsymmetrical flow conditions exist on the inlet side (such as entering the fan from a close-coupled 90° elbow or an occlusion created by the motor-drive), the tonal components of blade-frequency noise may increase by as much as 10 dB. In a typical HVAC application, the normal presence of these annoying tonal components dictates the need to consider the installation of high-efficiency sound attenuators on both the inlet and discharge sides of the fan. Actually, the use of high-efficiency sound attenuators and/or ductlining to control the transmission of noise at the blade-passage frequency is really not an option but a requirement in most HVAC applications of vaneaxial fans. The type and extent of other noise control requirements will be governed by the entrance and exit geometry in the region near the fan. A worst-case situation results if the flow enters the fan from a close-coupled 90° elbow or if the drive-motor and its mounting system happens to be located on the inlet side of the fan, thus creating an obstruction resulting in a loss of flow symmetry. Most, but unfortunately not all, manufacturers of vaneaxial equipment locate the drive-motor on the discharge side of the fan, or out of the airstream, to avoid disturbing the symmetry of the inlet flow.

The characteristic shape of the air performance curve of a typical vaneaxial fan has a pronounced knee to the left of the peak efficiency point, as illustrated in Figure 4-3. The system resistance curve, (c), intersects the fan curve in this undesirable knee region

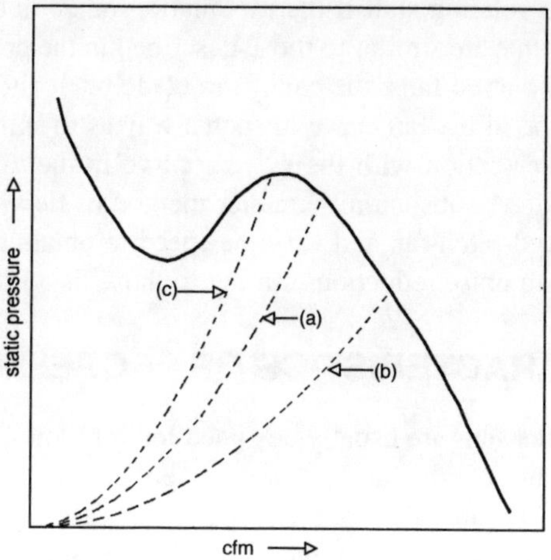

FIGURE 4-3 Characteristic air performance curve of a typical vaneaxial fan. The system resistance curve, (a), intersects the fan curve in the region of peak efficiency. The region between curves (a) and (b) is the range of normal fan selection. Operation in the region of curve (c), or farther to the left, will cause the fan to stall or surge.

where fan operation becomes unstable and rotating stall occurs. Acoustically, the rotating stall is characterized by a substantial increase in the level of low-frequency noise and vibration, principally concentrated at about two-thirds the fan rpm/60. Typically, this stall frequency will occur between 15 Hz and 30 Hz in most HVAC vaneaxial fan applications.

The system resistance curve, (a), intersects the fan curve in the region of peak efficiency, the quietest point of operation on the fan curve. The normal selection range lies between curves (a) and (b). Operation farther out on the fan curve beyond (b) results in an increased noise level in the mid- and high-frequency range of the sound spectrum; the farther to the right, the greater the increase.

FLOW MODULATION IN VARIABLE-VOLUME APPLICATIONS

There are typically two methods of flow control in variable-volume applications. The most common, but not the quietest, is to use a fan equipped with variable pitch blades and operated at a constant speed. Although a relatively high fan efficiency can be maintained during flow modulation, there is still the danger of shifting the fan into rotating stall if the modulation range is too great. The reasons for this are similar to those described in the previous section on forward-curved fans; the change in blade pitch alters the characteristic shape of the fan curve in such a way as to shift the effective point of intersection with the system curve in the direction of the rotating stall. A substantially quieter method of flow modulation is to use a fixed-pitch fan and vary the speed to obtain the desired air volume, with noise reductions similar to those listed in Table 4-2.

NOISE CHARACTERISTICS OF PROPELLER FANS

Propeller fans are usually designed for very low-pressure applications (many operate at or near free delivery conditions) and can handle high-volume flow rates. Propeller fans are manufactured in a wide range of blade shapes and sizes. Typical applications are roof exhaust fans, makeup fans, localized ventilation, air-cooled condensing units, and in cooling towers.

The predominant acoustical energy produced by propeller fan equipment is normally concentrated in the region of the blade-passage frequency (number of fan blades times the rpm/60, Hz). Since there are typically only a few fan blades (3 to 7), and operating speeds seldom exceed about 1200 rpm, the blade-passage frequency usually occurs in the frequency region below 100 Hz. For example, the blade-frequency produced by typical propeller fans used in many air-cooled condensing units is in the neighborhood of 80 Hz. The air performance of propeller fans is similar in many respects to that of vaneaxial fans, as illustrated in Figure 4-3. Because of the pronounced knee in the characteristic curve, it is very easy to induce a rotating stall in a propeller fan if the pressure rise across the fan exceeds about one inch, w.g.

In general, low-frequency acoustical energy below 100 Hz is very difficult to attenuate with any type of sound absorptive treatment. Even sound attenuators optimized to perform in the low-frequency region are not a practical option in many applications. This is because propeller fans are typically designed to operate close to free delivery conditions, and the added flow resistance of a sound attenuator frequently results in an unacceptable reduction in fan performance, as well as an increase in noise level that tends to offset the effect of the sound attenuator.

For example, in many field installations where packaged sound attenuators have been installed in an attempt to quiet propeller fan equipment, it has been found that the aerodynamic performance lost, due to the added system resistance, is sufficient to require either an increase in the pitch of the fan blades or in the operating speed (or both) to regain the required air delivery. Because the noise produced by a propeller fan increases rapidly with either increased pitch or tip-speed, the incremental change required to restore airflow usually offsets the effectiveness of the added sound attenuators. A better solution is to replace the fan with one of a quieter design because there is considerable variation in the design of propeller fans for a given application and some operate significantly quieter than others.

SOUND RATING OF PROPELLER FANS

AMCA Standard 300-85, Reverberant Room Method for Sound Testing of Fans contains procedures for testing propeller fans mounted in several configurations. The data obtained may be expressed on an octave band or one-third octave-band basis in terms of sound power levels with respect to 10^{-12} watt. Thus, at least in theory, acoustical data ought to be available from manufacturers of propeller fans for their various designs and sizes. In reality, the available database is not very extensive.

This situation exists because there are so many variables in propeller fan size and design that the manufacturers tend to not invest in rating their entire line of available equipment but often rely instead on highly questionable estimates made by extrapolating data obtained from a limited number of actual tests on fans, not necessarily of the same size or geometrically similar. Therefore, the design engineer should view the data supplied by a manufacturer of propeller fans with skepticism—unless they are known to have been obtained from tests on the actual fan in question.

There is also further cause for skepticism if the blade frequency (where most of the noise is concentrated) occurs in the region below 100 Hz. The procedure for qualification of a suitable laboratory test environment, in accordance with AMCA 300-85, is not applicable below 100 Hz. Therefore, if the fan blade-passage frequency lies below 100 Hz (which it almost always does), any available data are likely unreliable.

LOW-FREQUENCY NOISE ASSOCIATED WITH BELT DRIVES

Only very recently has it been recognized that not all of the low-frequency noise attributable to fan operation is of aerodynamic origin (Blazier 1993). Another prominent source has been traced to the dynamic mechanical forces produced by the belt-drive geometry in the fan assembly. The problem is most pronounced in packaged air-handling equipment where the belt-drive components and fan bearings typically are mounted in a frame that is structurally common with the fan housing in order to conserve space and reduce cost.

Frequently, the sheet metal gauge of the fan housing is so light that the side sheets are actually braced by angle struts anchored to the frame of the drive system to control "ballooning" at the operating static pressure. Consequently, the result of this cost and space-saving geometry is that all the dynamic forces produced by the belt-drive system are directly coupled to the side panels of the fan housing, which in turn are driven like the cone of a loudspeaker, thus radiating very low-frequency acoustical noise into the connected ductwork.

The frequency range, where a majority of this low-frequency energy is concentrated, is the region of 16 Hz to 32 Hz and is virtually impossible to control without substantial stiffening and lagging of the external ductwork. Therefore, in selecting packaged equipment for an acoustically sensitive application, it is important to specify that the fan/drive assembly be structurally independent of the fan housing.

REFERENCES

Blazier, W.E., Jr. 1993. Control of low-frequency noise in HVAC air-handling equipment and systems. *ASHRAE Transactions* 99(2): 1031-1036.

ISO. 1975. *ISO 532, Acoustics—Method for calculating loudness level*, Appendices A and B. Geneva: International Organization for Standardization.

Chapter 5
Central-Station Air-Handling Units

by *Charles Ebbing and Warren Blazier*

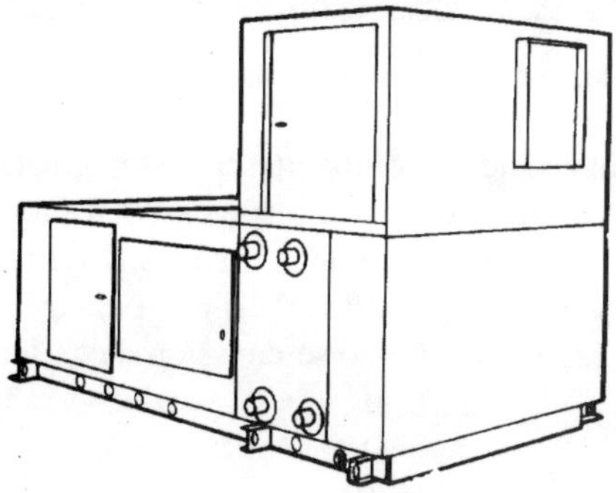

OVERVIEW

Central-station air-handling units (AHUs) are *packaged units*[1] that contain one or more fans to supply air to the conditioned space. Fan wheels are usually forward curved, backward inclined, or backward inclined airfoil centrifugal. Various internal accessories are used to filter, heat or cool the air, and control humidity. These units are usually located in mechanical equipment rooms or outdoors in rooftop-type applications.

NOISE CHARACTERISTICS OF CENTRAL-STATION AIR-HANDLING UNITS

Broad-band noise is generated at the fan wheel by the air turbulence and vortices and eddies created at the edge of each blade in a

1. Units can be shipped as an assembly, a "packaged unit," or be "built-up" from components.

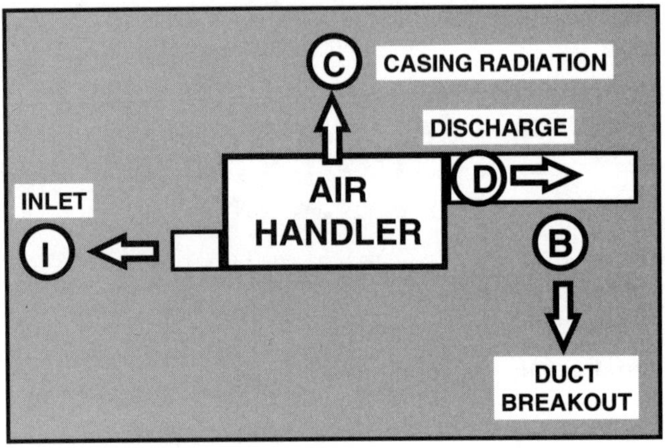

FIGURE 5-1 Noise sources of an air handler and discharge ductwork.

random manner; the higher the tip speed, the greater the sound generated. In addition, each time a blade passes a stationary support, or protuberance, in the airstream, an impulse noise is produced resulting in a tonal component called the blade-passage frequency.

Figure 5-1 shows the noise emission paths for an air-handling unit.

SOUND PATHS

Discharge Sound Path

Discharge sound is the sound that travels through the downstream ductwork, and it is delivered to the space along with the conditioned air. It is sometimes called *airborne sound.*

Casing Radiated Sound Path

This is sound that radiates from the air-handling unit casing and reaches the listener independently of that transmitted as airborne sound through the air supply ductwork. Typically, the casing radiated path is from the panels of the air-handling unit directly into the surrounding space.

Inlet Sound Path

Inlet sound radiates from the unit's return air opening and travels from the mechanical equipment room to the occupied space through either the return air ductwork or the equipment room walls.

Breakout Sound Path

Discharge sound travels through the downstream discharge ductwork causing it to vibrate the ductwork and radiate sound to the surrounding space.

FAN PERFORMANCE AND NOISE

Discharge Conditions Affecting Fan Noise

Poorly designed and installed discharge ductwork configurations will cause excessive turbulence and will affect fan performance and significantly increase system noise levels, especially at low frequencies as described in Chapter 4.

Fans used in central-station air handlers are typically tested and rated in the laboratory under ideal conditions at several fan speeds and over a range of operating points in the fan curve, as shown in Figure 5-2.

The configuration of ductwork used for these laboratory tests of fan equipment usually differs significantly from the actual configurations encountered in typical field installations. The uniform discharge velocity profile normally developed in the laboratory test setup is not likely achieved in the field because of disturbances caused by non-ideal flow conditions of connecting ductwork. For example, to obtain the same aerodynamic performance of the fan and the corresponding sound power level as when tested in the laboratory, straight ductwork downstream of the fan discharge for at

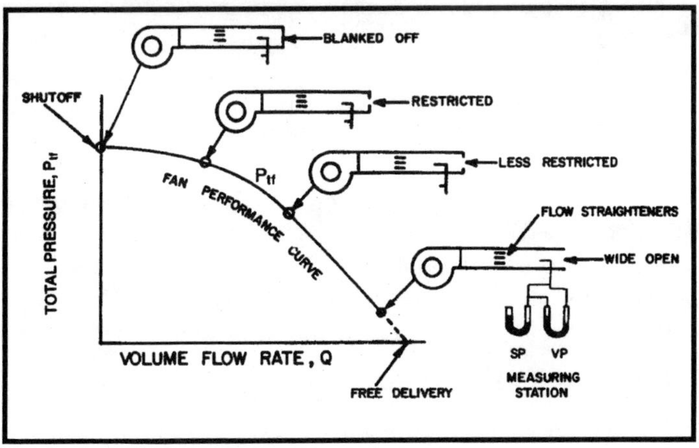

FIGURE 5-2 Method of developing a fan performance curve.

least several duct widths is essential. However, seldom does sufficient space exist to configure the ductwork in this manner. More commonly, it is necessary to install abrupt transitions and fittings in making connections to both the inlet and outlet. This results in compromises in fan performance and increased noise levels when compared to the manufacturer's laboratory test data (see Chapter 4 for more information).

Effect of Inlet Guide Vanes on Fan Noise

The use of inlet guide vanes is the most typical method of fan control in VAV systems. Inlet guide vanes are used with forward-curved fans, backward-inclined fans, and airfoil fans. However, even when the inlet vanes are in the full-open position, the disturbance in the air profile at the fan inlet produced by these vanes typically increases the operating noise level at least 5 dB because inserting the vanes changes the shape of the fan curve and likely reduces the fan efficiency, as described in Chapter 4.

Effect of Variable Frequency Drives on Fan Noise

Fan sound power levels decrease as fan speed is reduced. For instance, in a fixed system resistance duct system, at 50% of maximum fan speed, the operating sound level decreases by approximately 15 dB (Fragnito 1993), compared to that produced at 100% of full fan speed. Significant energy savings are also obtained at reduced fan speed because the horsepower required reduces as the cube of the speed ratio. For example, one-half of full speed requires only one-eighth of the horsepower corresponding to full-design airflow.

When using a variable frequency drive, it is important to determine the lowest anticipated operating fan speed because the static deflection of the vibration isolators supporting the fan equipment must be great enough to avoid exciting the resonance of the mounting system at the lowest fan speed. The reaction forces produced by an unbalanced fan decrease as the square of the fan speed. Thus, as a general rule, it is advisable to ensure that the ratio of minimum fan speed (rps) to the natural frequency of the isolation system (cps) is at least 2:1 to avoid magnifying fan vibration on its mounting system.

Riding the Fan Curve

When airflow is not modulated by inlet vanes or by a variable frequency drive in variable volume systems, the flow is modulated by the varying resistance of the air terminals. This mode of operation is known as "riding the fan curve" and can result in increased fan static pressure, and, thus, noise as flow is reduced in the selected range of fan operation. Also, noise caused by leaks in the ductwork or by high static pressure at the terminals will increase as the duct static pressure increases and could reach objectionable levels. Furthermore, riding the fan curve can result in unstable air delivery from the fan and a significant increase in low-frequency noise. This occurs if the range of modulation is such that the operating point on the fan curve is shifted to a region of rotating stall or surge. Forward-curved centrifugal or vaneaxial fans are particularly susceptible to this problem, as described in Chapter 4.

Other System Considerations

Blow-Through vs. Draw-Through Units

When fan noise is a major consideration, blow-through units offer significant advantages over draw-through units because the discharge sound power of a blow-through unit is usually substantially lower in comparison to a draw-through unit of the same capacity. However, the sound power radiated from the inlet side is usually similar for either unit configuration. The discharge sound power level is lower in a blow-through unit because of acoustical losses that occur as a result of the expansion at the fan outlet and the sound absorption that occurs within the downstream insulated coil section. In addition, the geometry of the opening in the discharge plenum of a blow-through unit can usually be designed to closely match the cross section of the dimensions of the main trunk duct, thus avoiding the excessive air turbulence and noise that typically occurs at fan-to-duct transitions of a draw-through unit.

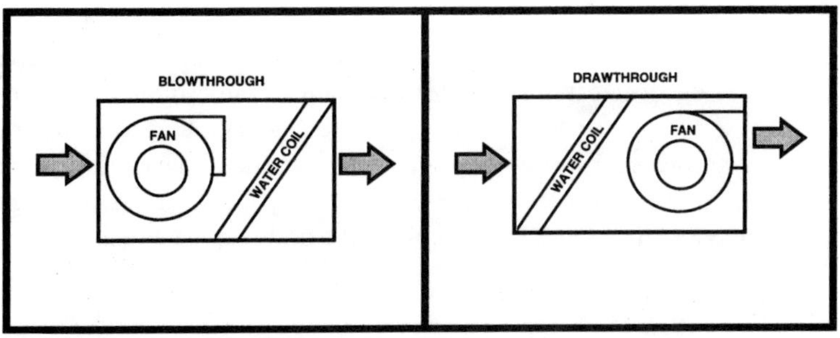

Figure 5-3 Arrangements of blow-through vs. draw-through air handlers.

Main Trunk Duct

The size and shape of the main building trunk duct is usually a result of the methodology used to design the duct system and the floor-to-floor height design of the building. For example, it is common practice to begin sizing the system at the air terminal that is furthest from the fan, making sure that there is sufficient static pressure to control and operate the air terminal in that location. The branch duct is sized at this point, and then either the static-regain method or the equal-friction method is used to size the remaining ductwork, working back to the mechanical equipment room. In sizing the main ducts, height restrictions dictated by the plenum space above the ceiling usually limit the available duct height. Consequently, the size of the duct is determined by the width necessary to meet the duct cross-sectional area required. The potential of encountering breakout noise problems in the region below the main ducts is significantly increased as these ducts become wider and have a larger aspect ratio.

Duct Transition Design Guidelines

Extreme care and caution should be exercised in the design and installation of transition fittings to the inlet or discharge of air handlers. Experience has shown that poorly designed and installed transition fittings are a major cause of many low-frequency noise problems associated with duct rumble. The discharge connection from an air-handling unit should ideally be a straight duct. If a transition fitting is required, the ideal design would utilize a slope of no more than 1 in 7 (8 degrees) (Fragnito 1993). However, for a two-dimensional expansion, a slope of no more than 1 in 4 (14 degrees) may be acceptable if the discharge velocity does not exceed 2000 ft/min.

When the contained angle of the transition fitting exceeds these angles, the air does not cling to the sides of the duct and flow separation occurs, resulting in the formation of large turbulent eddies. These turbulent eddies create pressure fluctuations and also large system pressure losses, both of which generate unwanted low-frequency noise. Whenever the fitting is expanded in two different planes and the slopes are excessive, the problem is more acute.

Aerodynamic Noise of Duct Fittings

It is possible to estimate the resulting sound level in occupied spaces due simply to fan noise by using the algorithms for the acoustical attenuation of path elements developed by ASHRAE (1991), but the incremental sound power level contributed by flow-induced noise generated by duct elements and fittings cannot be reliably estimated because these relationships have yet to be developed and documented. Therefore, the best alternative for minimizing the effects of flow-induced noise by duct elements and fittings is to use good aerodynamic design practices to avoid excessive duct velocities, flow direction changes, and rapid duct expansions.

MANUFACTURERS' SOUND RATING PROCEDURES AND PRACTICES FOR CENTRAL-STATION AIR HANDLERS

SOUND STANDARDS AND DATA AVAILABILITY

Draft Air Conditioning and Refrigeration Institute Standard 260P

AMCA Standard 300-85 is the basis for *Draft ARI Standard 260P, Sound Rating of Ducted Air-Moving Equipment.* This draft standard outlines procedures for rating the sound power levels of discharge, inlet, and casing-radiated noise for all ducted HVAC equipment, including packaged air-handling units.

Air Moving and Control Association Standard 300-85

AMCA Standard 300-85, Reverberant Room Method for Sound Testing of Fans, is the test standard most frequently used by the industry for obtaining sound power level data for stand-alone or built-up fan equipment. Although packaged air-handling units are not under the purview of the AMCA program, industry practice has been to use the closest relevant test standard if no actual test standard exists for the equipment being evaluated. Thus, the AMCA Standard 300-85 has become the defacto procedure used by most manufacturers when testing inlet, discharge, and casing radiated noise of air-handling units. This is also the standard most consulting engineers reference in specifications.

ASHRAE 68-1986 and AMCA 330-86 (In-Duct Fan Sound Power Testing)

These standards establish an in-duct test method for determining the sound power level of a fan. The procedure is based on measuring the sound pressure level in the airstream of either the supply duct or return duct. The sound power level is determined from the sound pressure measurements based on the cross-sectional area of the test duct. Note that this is a combined ASHRAE/AMCA standard. For air handlers, the in-duct test method is an alternative to the reverberation-room test method described above, but it is currently used mainly for research purposes.

Sound Test Overview

Figures 17-2 through 17-4 in Chapter 17 show examples of typical air-handling test setups for measuring the discharge, inlet, and casing-radiated noise using ARI Standard 260P.[2] In Figure 17-2 (discharge noise), the unit is installed outside the room and the discharge side is connected to the reverberant room to measure discharge noise. In Figure 17-3 (inlet noise), the inlet side is connected to the reverberant room to measure only the inlet noise. In Figure 17-4 (casing-radiated noise[3]), the unit is located in the reverberant room and heavy-gage, stiffened, and lagged ductwork is used to transfer the inlet and discharge noise to the exterior of the test room so that the main noise radiated to the reverberation is from the casing of the unit.

For all three tests, the unit is loaded aerodynamically as quietly as possible to simulate the static pressure rise the unit will encounter during application.

Low-frequency sound data

The meaningful determination of sound power levels in the 16 Hz and 31.5 Hz octave bands requires a reverberation room substantially larger than 10,000 ft^3 (300 m^3).[4] Therefore, most manufacturers' sound power level data do not include data at these frequencies because of the costs involved in the construction of large rooms and the difficulties encountered in qualifying a test room of such a large physical size. Current ANSI and ISO reverberation room standards specify measurements down to 100 Hz.[5]

Field noise problems that often occur in the 16 Hz, 31.5 Hz,

---

2. The reverberant room wall construction must be capable of safely withstanding the room pressurization from this test.
3. The accepted term "casing-radiated" radiated noise may be a bit misleading to some readers. This is the noise radiating from the panels or external surfaces of the air handler.
4. Most industry reverberant rooms are less than 10,000 ft^3 (300 m^3) volume.

and 63 Hz octave bands are often caused by system effects that can only be minimized by exercising good aerodynamic design practices in the design of ductwork and the appropriate selection of a fan that will be stable and operate efficiently in the connected system with its anticipated system effects.[6]

Reference sound source

Most ARI and AMCA test standards are based on use of a calibrated reference sound source in determining the sound power level of a device under test, such as a fan. The reference sound source, also known as a standard source, is a small direct-drive fan wheel[7] that operates without a fan scroll. This fan is designed and built to strict specifications that result in a stable sound power level output from 63 Hz[8] to 8000 Hz. The reference source is designed to have a relatively uniform broad-band sound power level output in each octave band.

To determine the sound power level of an unknown source, sound pressure measurements are first made with the reference sound source operating in the test room. Then, the reference source is turned off and the measurements are repeated with the unknown source in operation. Because the sound power level of the reference source is a known value, the differences in measured sound pressure levels between the reference source and unknown source represent differences in the sound power level between the two. Thus, the sound power level of the unknown source can be deduced by adding these differences to the sound power level of the reference source. This procedure for sound power level determination is known as the substitution method.

Data Availability

Most manufacturers provide sound power level data for discharge, inlet, and casing-radiated noise in octave bands, as illustrated in Table 5-1.

The greatest problem is with the quality and, hence, reliability

5. ARI has recently released qualification requirements in ARI Standard 280 for the 63 Hz octave band.
6. Manufacturers' data does not reflect the presence of these system effects.
7. See Chapter 17 for more information on reference sound sources.
8. This octave band contains a narrow-band rotating stall component in some existing reference sound source designs that can introduce an error in the sound power determination.

TABLE 5-1
Central-Station Air Handlers Data Summary

Oct. Band Range Hz	Most Important Bands	Data Rating Points
Usually 63 Hz - 8000 Hz	31.5 Hz - 250 Hz	Usually Over a Range of Flow and Pressure

of the data, which varies widely within the industry. The data can come from several sources:

- Measured data obtained over a range of operating points and often regressed into a set of equations that permits the estimation of sound power levels at any point within the range of the measured data.
- Measured data at an unspecified operating point for the unit in question.
- Calculated data based on old ASHRAE algorithms that are no longer considered reliable (Reynolds and Bledsoe 1991).
- Estimated data that are based upon assumptions and have no basis in fact.

Most manufacturers measure data in one-third octave bands but only report octave-band sound power information as currently required by the industry. However, one-third octave-band information is necessary to detect the presence of pure tones. This can usually be obtained upon request from many manufacturers of air-handling equipment.

Variability of Data

As with any laboratory test procedure, there are always measurement uncertainties to be taken into account when reporting or using manufacturers' sound data. The uncertainties in the low-frequency acoustical data using measurement procedures, such as those specified by ARI 260P, are dependent upon the physical size of the reverberation test chamber. The larger the size of the test chamber, the less the uncertainty is in the data reported in the low-frequency octave bands. Experience indicates that the uncertainties in accuracy of measured data,[9] as listed in Table 5-2, should be considered when applying current manufacturers' test data to an HVAC system design.

9. It is assumed that the reverberation room meets the applicable reverberation room standards.

TABLE 5-2
Estimated Variability of Product Sound Power Data Due to Measurement Uncertainties and Production Quality Control and in Octave Bands Most Affected by System Effects and Point-of-Fan Operation (Shaded Areas)

Air-Handling Units						
Octave Mid-Band Frequency	**Measurement Uncertainty of Std. Test Procedure[a] dB**	**Repeatability of Test Data[b] dB**	**Production Variability[c] dB**	**Cumulative Uncer-tainty Due To All Previous Factors[d] dB**	**Variability of Random Sample *re* Catalog[e] dB**	**Bands Most Affected by System Effects and Point-of-Fan Operation[f]**
31.5	Data not available	Data not available	Data not available	Data not available	Data not available	+5 to15 dB
63	± 4 dB[g]	± 2 dB	± 4 dB	± 6 dB	+6, -0	+5 to15 dB
125	± 3 dB	± 1 dB	± 3 dB	± 4 dB	+5, -0	+5 to15 dB
250	± 2 dB	± 1 dB	± 3 dB	± 4 dB	+3, -0	+0 to 5 dB
500-4000	± 1.5 dB	± 1 dB	± 3 dB	± 4 dB	+3, -0	+0 to 5 dB
8000	± 3 dB	± 0.5 dB	± 3 dB	± 4 dB	+3, -0	+0 to 5 dB

a. Standard deviation of octave band data per ISO 3741.
b. Repetitive testing of same unit in same laboratory.
c. Subject to manufacturing tolerances permitted in production quality-control.
d. Based on the square root of the sum of the squares of all uncertainties.
e. Published catalog data are not customarily derived from a statistical sampling of production units but usually are determined by testing a prototype. Thus, the results of testing random production samples would tend to exceed those published by the manufacturer.
f. See Chapter 1 for discussion of the effects of system effects on installed noise levels.
g. ARI has recently completed *ARI Standard 280, Requirements for the Qualification of Reverberant Rooms in the 63 Hz Octave Band*. This standard outlines the qualification requirements for the 63 Hz octave band.

CUSTOM AIR-HANDLING UNIT DATA

Manufacturers' sound power level data for custom air-handling units are usually calculated (not measured) levels generated by proprietary computer programs. The programs estimate the inlet, discharge, and casing-radiated sound power levels based on the proposed AHU design. The programs take into consideration the following characteristics: the unit configuration, the sound transmission and absorption properties of the proposed panel construction, the sizes and locations of the inlet and discharge openings, and the sound power levels of the AHU fan as determined by AMCA 300-85.

In general, these programs assume that the fan(s) inside the AHUs generate the same sound power levels when installed in the unit as they do in the optimal configuration employed in the AMCA 300-85 test setup. This is not a valid assumption because the close proximity of the cabinet panels, fan support structure, and other components (e.g., inlet vanes) will increase the fan's sound power levels above those measured using AMCA 300-85.

In addition, the algorithms used in the estimation programs typically include engineering estimates (which can vary significantly from manufacturer to manufacturer) of the panels' sound transmission loss and sound absorption properties. This is particularly true of the 63 Hz octave band for which virtually no laboratory test data is available. (The test standards, ASTM E90 and ASTM C423, do not requisite testing at frequencies below 100 Hz.) Because of these inherent problems, custom AHU discharge, inlet, and casing-radiated sound power levels derived from computer programs should be used with caution. The preferred method of determining AHU sound power levels is via direct laboratory measurements using AMCA 300-85 or ARI Draft Standard 260P.

RECOMMENDED DESIGN AND INSTALLATION PRACTICES FOR CENTRAL-STATION AIR-HANDLING UNITS

SIZE AND TYPE

1. Either oversizing or undersizing fans produces more noise than when properly sized. Oversizing often results in excessive low-frequency noise below 125 Hz, which is difficult to attenuate with passive sound attenuators. Undersizing results in an increase in noise but in a higher frequency region that can be compensated for by adding duct lining or passive attenuators.
2. A blow-through unit produces significantly less discharge noise than a draw-through unit because the coil and accessory section on the downstream side of the fan acts as a plenum that reduces the level of low- and mid-frequency noise.

LOCATION

1. Locate the air-handling unit next to areas that are not noise sensitive, such as restrooms, copy rooms, storage areas,

stairwells, and other spaces where ambient level can be relatively high.

2. To provide adequate support for vibration isolation, locate the unit over vertical structural building supports. Do not locate units close to the center of unsupported floor spans.
3. Keep duct velocities as low as possible. Table 5-3 lists the maximum air velocities recommended to avoid excessive airflow-related noise in most noncritical applications.
4. Locate the first 20 ft of discharge duct over spaces that can tolerate more low-frequency noise.

TABLE 5-3
Recommended Maximum Duct Velocity and Minimum Duct Gauge

Max. Duct Width (in.)	Max. Recommended Air Velocity (fpm)	Min. Recommended Duct Gage
12-36	2000	24
36-48	1800	22
48-72	1600	20
72-96	1400	18

Note: See also *1995 ASHRAE Handbook—HVAC Applications*, Chapter 43, for other guidelines pertaining to duct velocity recommendations.

DUCT DESIGN

Use full-radiused elbow with turning vanes for first turn of supply duct. Elbow locations should follow the ASHRAE guidelines.

1. The stiffness of the ductwork is very important in the control of low-frequency breakout noise. When discharge ductwork is installed over noise sensitive spaces, use heavy gauge sheet metal or round ductwork to minimize low-frequency duct breakout noise.
2. Exterior stiffening of the ductwork may also be required. Round ductwork, as illustrated in Figure 5-4, radiates significantly less noise at low frequencies. The heavier the duct gage, the less the breakout noise. Changing from a rectangular 24-gage duct to a rectangular 16-gage duct can reduce breakout noise by 6 dB in the 31.5 Hz and 63 Hz bands.
3. Duct stiffness of a rectangular duct can be significantly improved by increasing the stiffness of the duct between the angle brackets by attaching drywall, as in Figure 5-5.

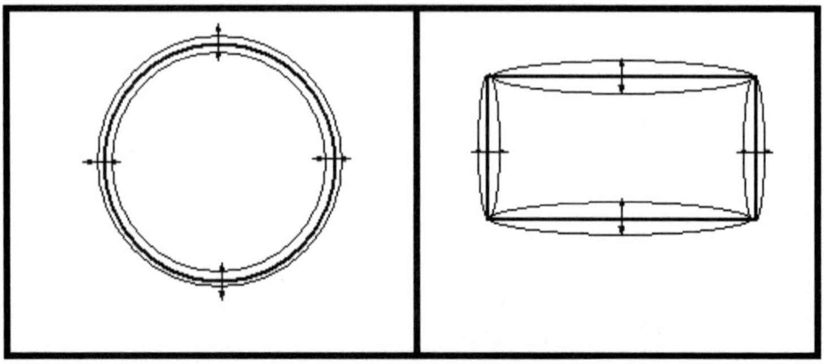

FIGURE 5-4 Round ductwork is much stiffer and harder to vibrate at low frequencies than rectangular ductwork.

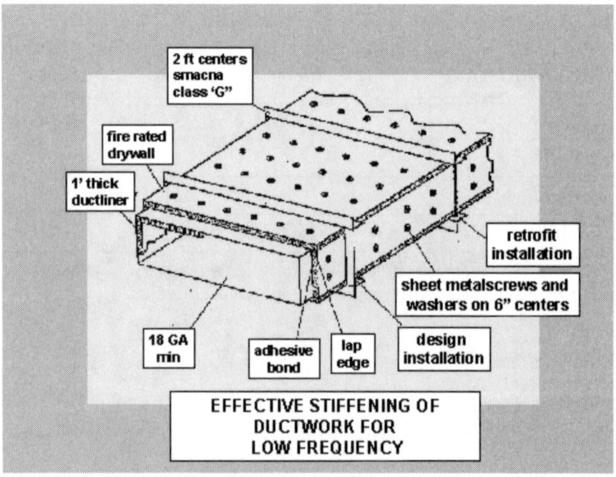

FIGURE 5-5 Increasing the stiffness of the duct by attaching drywall to reduce breakout noise (ASHRAE 1995).

4. Duct design and layout, along with construction and installation practices, should follow the guidelines outlined by ASHRAE (ASHRAE 1995) and as specified by SMACNA standards (SMACNA 1981, 1985). It is also good practice to maintain small aspect ratios in the design of ductwork.

Note: Passive sound attenuators in the lengths normally available are generally ineffective in attenuating noise in the frequency region of 63 Hz and below. Therefore, they offer little benefit in the solution of problems involving low-frequency noise problems. Therefore, care should be exercised in ductwork design to prevent low-frequency noise problems.

Vibration Isolation

It is advisable to vibration-isolate air-handling units in any location within a building structure. However, both the method of vibration isolation and the degree of isolation efficiency depend upon factors such as equipment location and characteristics of the building structure. For guidance in the selection of an appropriate vibration isolation system, refer to Table 42 in Chapter 43 of the *1995 ASHRAE Handbook—Applications*.

SUGGESTED NOISE SPECIFICATIONS

Estimate the Maximum Allowable Sound Power

By using the acoustic calculation procedure outlined in Chapter 43 of the *ASHRAE Handbook*, the designer can estimate and specify the maximum allowable sound power of central-station air-handling units in each octave band.

The manufacturer of air-handling units must accept responsibility for meeting the specified sound power level of the supplied air-handling equipment (see Table 5-4); however, it is not possible for the manufacturer to accept responsibility for, or guarantee that, the specified room sound pressure levels in occupied spaces will be met when the HVAC system is placed into operation. There are too many factors that influence the sound level in an occupied space that are beyond the control of the equipment manufacturer. Such factors include building design, materials and furnishings, duct system design, and installation. Although sound pressure levels can be measured in the occupied space with reasonable accuracy, it is rarely possible to demonstrate in the field that the manufacturer's submitted sound power level data are not as specified.

Table 5-4
Sample Air-Handling Specifications

Sound Specifications				**Maximum L_w Values in dB *re* 1 Picowatt Octave Band Center Frequency in Hz**							
Mark	cfm	tsp	Source	63	125	250	500	1k	2k	4k	8k
AHU-2	7000	4.5	Discharge								
	7000	4.5	Inlet								
	7000	4.5	Casing Radiation								

The only reliable basis upon which to establish compliance with the specified levels is a witness-test at the manufacturer's facility prior to shipment of the equipment performed in accordance with ARI 260P, as previously described.

Noise Specifications

All air-handling units listed in this schedule shall have been tested in accordance with ARI Standard 260, Sound Rating of Ducted Air-Moving Equipment. *When operating at the operating points shown, the values of sound power level* (L_W) *shall not exceed those scheduled in Table 5-4.*

APPLICATION OF MANUFACTURERS' DATA

Having received the manufacturer's sound power level data for discharge, inlet, and casing-radiated noise, the estimated sound pressure levels in the occupied spaces can be determined using the methods outlined in the most current *ASHRAE Handbook—Applications*.

REFERENCES

ASHRAE. 1991. *1991 ASHRAE handbook—HVAC applications.* Atlanta: American Society of Heating, Refrigerating and Air-Conditioning Engineers, Inc.

ASHRAE. 1995. *1995 ASHRAE handbook—HVAC applications.* Atlanta: American Society of Heating, Refrigerating and Air-Conditioning Engineers, Inc.

Fragnito, D. 1993. Air-handling equipment acoustics. *Carrier Corporation Application Manual 811-589.*

Reynolds, D., and J. Bledsoe. 1991. *Algorithms for HVAC acoustics.* Atlanta: American Society of Heating, Refrigerating and Air-Conditioning Engineers, Inc.

SMACNA. 1981. *HVAC duct system design*, 2d ed. Vienna, Va: Sheet Metal and Air-Conditioning Contractors' Association.

SMACNA. 1985. *HVAC duct construction standards.* Vienna, Va: Sheet Metal and Air-Conditioning Contractors' Association.

Chapter 6
Commercial Packaged HVAC Equipment

by *Charles Ebbing and Warren Blazier*

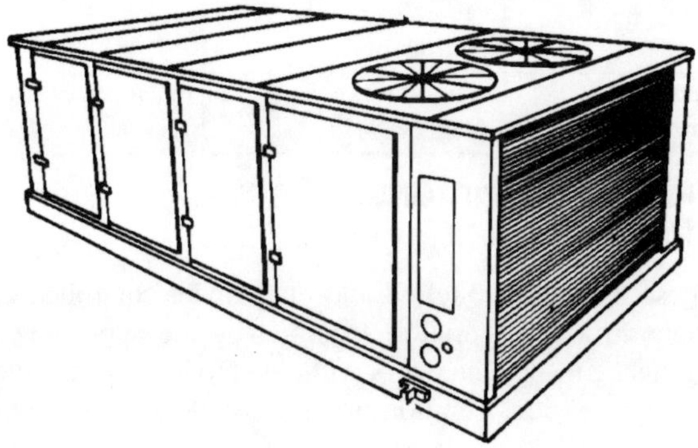

OVERVIEW

Commercial packaged HVAC equipment includes rooftop units, vertical air conditioners, water source heat pumps (WSHP), and packaged terminal air conditioners (PTACS). Rooftop units range from 1 ton to 11 tons for small rooftops and from 12 tons up to over 200 tons for large rooftops. Vertical air-conditioner product sizes range from 3 tons to 60 tons, water source heat pump product sizes range from 0.5 tons to 20 tons. Packaged terminal air-conditioner sizes range from 0.5 tons to 1.5 tons.

NOISE CHARACTERISTICS OF DUCTED PACKAGED EQUIPMENT

The noise sources in these products are the compressors and fans illustrated in Table 6-1. Noise travels to the receiver by various paths.

TABLE 6-1
Indoor and Outdoor Noise Sources in Packaged Products

Packaged Product	Indoor Sources	Outdoor Sources
Rooftop Units	· Supply fan discharge · Return air fan · Exhaust fan · Outside air intake · Leakage through roof curb to space below · Sound from bottom of unit transmitted through roof	· Condenser fan · Compressor · Exhaust and (discharge) · Outside air intake
Vertical Air Conditioner	· Evaporator fan · Compressor	
Water Source Heat Pump	· Evaporator fan · Compressor	
Package Terminal Air Conditioner	· Evaporator fan · Compressor	· Condenser fan

DISCHARGE CONDITIONS AFFECTING FAN PERFORMANCE

These products are tested and rated under controlled laboratory conditions in a configuration specified by the applicable ARI test standard using in-line ductwork without elbows or tees, which differs from the typical configuration in field installations. Poorly designed or installed inlet/discharge ductwork affects the unit performance and also creates additional noise not present in the manufacturer's equipment sound ratings. Therefore, laboratory performance ratings of airflow, static pressure, and sound power will not usually be duplicated in a field installation unless the configuration of inlet and discharge connecting ductwork approaches the laboratory conditions. For example, as illustrated in Figure 6-1, most field installations use tees and elbow transitions, close coupled to the fan intake or discharge; these significantly affect not only the fan performance but increase the noise produced as well by as much as 5 dB to 15 dB.

MANUFACTURERS' SOUND RATING PROCEDURES AND PRACTICES FOR DUCTED PACKAGED PRODUCTS

SOUND STANDARDS AND DATA AVAILABILITY

Industry Trade Association

The Air Conditioning and Refrigeration Institute (ARI) devel-

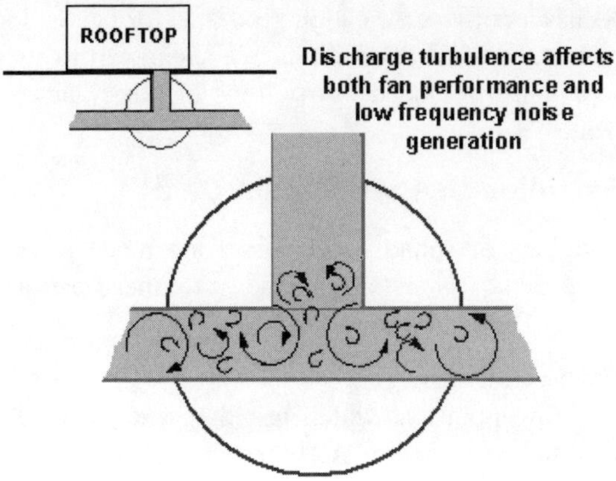

FIGURE 6-1 Discharge turbulence effects.

ops the standards for rating packaged equipment as listed in Table 6-2. These include ratings for both indoor and outdoor noise. The data used for sound rating are determined in reverberant room test facilities[1] over a range of flow and static pressure conditions (indoor data) and for the ARI test conditions (outdoor data). These indoor and outdoor ratings are usually determined with the equipment operating at standard operating conditions as specified in the applicable standard. The indoor ratings for PTACS are also often available from many manufacturers at each available fan speed.

TABLE 6-2
Applicable ARI Standards for Packaged Products

Packaged Product	Indoor Test Standards	Outdoor Test Standards
Rooftop Units	ARI 260P	ARI 270 up to 10 tons ARI 370 above 10 tons
Vertical Air Conditioners	ARI 260P	(No outdoor sources)
Water Source Heat Pumps	ARI 260P	(No outdoor sources)
Packaged Terminal Air Conditioners[a,b]	ARI 300	

a. ARI Standard 300 refers to ARI Standard 350 for indoor noise, ARI Standard 270 for outdoor noise, and ASTM E90-85 to determine the sound transmission loss of the PTAC with the unit damper closed.

b. The ASTM E90-85 rating calculated with the PTAC unit is mounted in the test wall in accordance with the provisions of ASTM Standard E90-85 with the unit not running and with the damper closed. The rating is calculated using the area of the outside dimensions of that portion of the wall sleeve that penetrates the outer face of the wall.

1. See Chapter 17 for more details on reverberant room testing.

ARI has a noise certification program[2] for the outdoor noise of rooftop units, but ARI does not have a sound certification program for indoor noise produced by rooftops or other ducted, packaged equipment.

Test Facilities Used to Obtain Data

All ratings of sound power level are made in reverberation rooms. Typical equipment arrangements for these tests are shown in Chapter 17, "Test Procedures."

Data rating points

The rating points at which test data are obtained for indoor noise are either specified by ARI thermal performance standards or, when not so specified, are chosen by the equipment manufacturer. Sound power ratings are typically available for a range of airflows, static pressures, and at several fan speeds.

Sound ratings and availability of data

Sound ratings for ducted packaged equipment are expressed in terms of sound power level. These are summarized in Table 6-3. The indoor rating is expressed in decibels (dB) at the octave-band center frequencies extending from 125 Hz to 8000 Hz. The outdoor rating is expressed as an A-weighted sound power level in decibels. Availability of data is generally better for the larger tonnage ducted, packaged equipment (above 12 tons). In many cases, indoor data are not available for smaller tonnage packaged equipment.

TABLE 6-3
Packaged Products Data Summary

<table>
<tr><th>Product</th><th>Outdoor Rating</th><th>Indoor Rating</th></tr>
<tr><td>Rooftop Units</td><td>A-weighted sound power level in decibels</td><td rowspan="3">Sound power level in octave bands
63 Hz - 8000 Hz
Usually over a range of flow and pressure</td></tr>
<tr><td>WSHP</td><td>N/A</td></tr>
<tr><td>Vertical Air Conditioners</td><td>N/A</td></tr>
<tr><td>PTAC</td><td>A-weighted sound power level in decibels</td><td>Sound power level at each fan speed</td></tr>
</table>

2. ARI has sound certification programs for air terminals, fan coil units, and outdoor condensing units. Participating manufacturers' units are sampled on a regular basis and tested in an independent lab.

Variability of Data

As with any laboratory test procedure, there are always measurement uncertainties to be taken into account when reporting data. The uncertainty in the low-frequency acoustical data using measurement procedures such as those specified by the ARI 260P[3] reverberant-room method are dependent on the physical size of the reverberant-room test chamber. The larger the size of the test chamber, the less the uncertainty in the measurements in the lower frequency octave bands. Experience indicates that uncertainties in the probable accuracy of measurements,[4] as shown in Table 6-4, should be considered when applying manufacturer's test data to an HVAC system design.

APPLICATION OF SOUND RATINGS OF DUCTED PACKAGED PRODUCTS TO BUILDING SYSTEMS

Good Design Practice for Noise Control

Size-Related Issues

1. Don't oversize or undersize capacity of rooftop, vertical air conditioners, or water-source heat pump units. Oversizing often results in excessive low-frequency noise from centrifugal fans. Undersizing increases high-frequency noise from centrifugal fans. This often happens when fan operation diversity is ignored or when other "design safety" factors are misused.
2. From a noise control standpoint, small ducted packaged units are usually easier to deal with than larger units. As unit size increases, more sound is concentrated adjacent to sensitive occupied spaces, and the potential for low-frequency duct breakout noise also increases significantly.
3. To avoid excessive noise in occupied spaces, do not locate water-source heat pump console units larger than 1.5 tons in small rooms of floor area less than 200 ft^2 (19 m^2).

Configuration-Related Issues to Minimize Noise Problems

1. Make certain that supply-air elbows connected to centrifugal fans turn in the same direction as the direction of fan rotation.

3. ARI 260P Draft Standard, Sound Rating of Ducted Air Moving and Conditioning Equipment.
4. It is assumed that the reverberation room meets the current ANSI or ISO reverberation room standards.

TABLE 6-4
Estimated Variability of Product Sound Power Data Due to Measurement Uncertainties and Production Quality Control
The Octave Bands Most Affected by System Effects in the Application, which May Alter the Operating Point on the Fan Curve, are also Indicated (Shaded Areas).

Air-Handling Units						
Octave Mid-Band Frequency	Measurement Uncertainty of Std. Test Procedure[a] dB	Repeatability of Test Data[b] dB	Production Variability[c] dB	Cumulative Uncer-tainty Due To All Previous Factors[d] dB	Variability of Random Sample *re* Catalog[e] dB	Bands Most Affected by Fan Operat-ing Point and System Effects[f] dB
63	± 4 dB[g]	± 2 dB	± 4 dB	± 6 dB	+6, -0	+5 to15 dB
125	± 3 dB	± 1 dB	± 3 dB	± 4 dB	+5, -0	+5 to15 dB
250	± 2 dB	± 1 dB	± 3 dB	± 4 dB	+3, -0	+5 to15 dB
500-4000	± 1.5 dB	± 1 dB	± 3 dB	± 4 dB	+3, -0	+0 to 5 dB
8000	± 3 dB	± 0.5 dB	± 3 dB	± 4 dB	+3, -0	+0 to 5 dB

a. Standard deviation of octave band data per ISO 3741.
b. Repetitive testing of same unit in same laboratory.
c. Subject to manufacturing tolerances permitted in production quality-control.
d. Based on the square root of the sum of the squares of all uncertainties.
e. Published catalog data are not customarily derived from a statistical sampling of production units but usually are determined by testing a prototype. Thus, the results of testing random production samples would tend to exceed those published by the manufacturer.
f. See Chapter 4 for discussion of how system noise levels are affected by the point of operation on the fan curve.
g. ARI has recently completed *ARI Standard 280, Requirements for the Qualification of Reverberant Rooms in the 63 Hz Octave Band*. This standard outlines the qualification requirements for the 63 Hz octave band.

2. With rooftop units, a heating section incorporated downstream of the cooling coil can serve as a discharge plenum and help reduce rumble.
3. When internal vibration isolation is provided by the equipment manufacturer for fans and compressors, the installer is advised to read the installation instructions to determine if the isolators have been bolted down or bypassed for shipment and need to be released. A properly vibration-isolated component must move freely when pushed by hand or foot.
4. While some manufacturers provide vibration isolation for compressors and fans, it may not be sufficiently effective on structures with long roof spans. In these cases, external

isolation is required. Consult Table 42, Chapter 43, *1995 ASHRAE Handbook—Applications* for specific recommendations.

Duct-Related Issues to Minimize Noise Problems

1. Minimize flow obstructions such as isolation dampers and tee splits in the ductwork near the fan.
2. The stiffness of the initial ductwork is very important in the control of low-frequency breakout noise. Using heavy gauge sheet metal, stiffened, or round ductwork is recommended downstream from the main duct extending from the fan to the first noise sensitive space.
3. Make sure that all fan discharge duct connections are made with flexible connections. Flexible connections should be made inside the roof curb for rooftop units.
4. For rectangular ductwork, use full radiused, equal dimensioned elbow with turning vanes for first turn in fan supply duct.
5. Line ductwork from inlet and outlet of fan to at least the first noise sensitive occupied space, or alternately, use sound attenuators carefully selected to minimize system effects.
6. Keep duct velocities (Ebbing et al. 1978) as low as possible. Table 6-5 shows the maximum flow that can be used without concern for excessive regenerated noise. Elbows connected to rooftop units, vertical air conditioners, and water-source heat pumps should have 1 in. thick duct liner unless greater noise control requires the use of properly designed elbow silencers.
7. Extend and line return air ductwork.

TABLE 6-5
Recommended Maximum Duct Velocity and Minimum Duct Gauge

Max. Duct Width (in.)	Max. Recommended Air Velocity (fpm)	Min. Recommended Duct Gage
12-36	2000	24
36-48	1800	22
48-72	1600	20
72-96	1400	18

Location Issues

1. Side-takeoff rooftop units produce less low-frequency noise in the supply ductwork than downward discharge units because the runout of ductwork above the roof allows a significant portion of the low-frequency sound to radiate from the duct sidewalls before entering the occupied space.
2. Locate units over nonsensitive spaces. When applying downward discharge units as shown in Figure 6-2, site the rooftop unit above bathrooms or other noncritical space to permit most of the low-frequency noise to radiate into spaces where excessive low-frequency noise can be tolerated. Whenever feasible, ducted-packaged equipment should be installed adjacent to or above nonsensitive occupied spaces such as restrooms, equipment rooms, storage areas, copy rooms, unoccupied areas, or other locations where the ambient noise level is already relatively high. Always attempt to avoid locations adjacent to or above conference rooms, private offices, classrooms, executive offices, libraries, and other noise-sensitive spaces.

Other Issues

1. Make sure that all water, electrical, and duct connections to water-source heat pump units are made with flexible connections.
2. Vertical water source heat pump units (Schaffer 1991) should be located in closets. Supply and return ducts

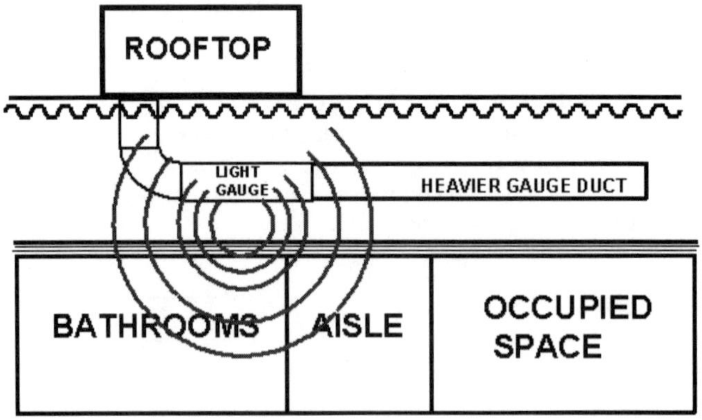

FIGURE 6-2 Applying downward discharging rooftop units.

should be lined with 1 in. thick ductliner. Closet doors should be gasketed for 3 ton and larger vertical units.

Source Noise Control Options

Outdoor Noise from Rooftop Units

1. Outdoor noise is produced by fans and compressors. Since few practical noise-control options exist for the outdoor noise sources, it is critical that units be located in such a manner as to minimize the noise impact on nearby noise-sensitive receivers. In some situations, manufacturers and users have added "slip-on" noise shields to the compressors. Unfortunately, these are only beneficial when the dominant outdoor noise is radiating from the compressor case. This is seldom the principal problem, and noise shields for compressors are often found to be of limited value.
2. Noise barriers can be used to control noise radiated in specific directions. A barrier should be no closer than that recommended by the manufacturer to the unit because the thermal capacity of the unit can be significantly affected by discharge air recirculation. For distances from the unit to the barrier closer than 6 ft and for barrier heights extending beyond the top of the fan discharge, it is recommended that the manufacturer be contacted to determine whether air recirculation is likely to affect the product performance.

Indoor Noise from Ducted Packaged Units

Supply noise path noise control

1. Make certain that supply ductwork follows the SMACNA guidelines for duct stiffness (SMACNA 1985). Ductwork can be externally stiffened, as shown in Figure 6-3. It is also desirable to partition or split large ductwork into smaller branches since smaller ductwork is both stiffer and a poorer radiator of low-frequency noise than large ductwork.
2. Line ductwork with at least 1 in. (25 mm) thick[5] duct liner from both the inlet and outlet of a fan to at least the first

5. Use 2 in. (50 mm) thick lining, if possible, when avoiding low-frequency rumble problems are a prime consideration.

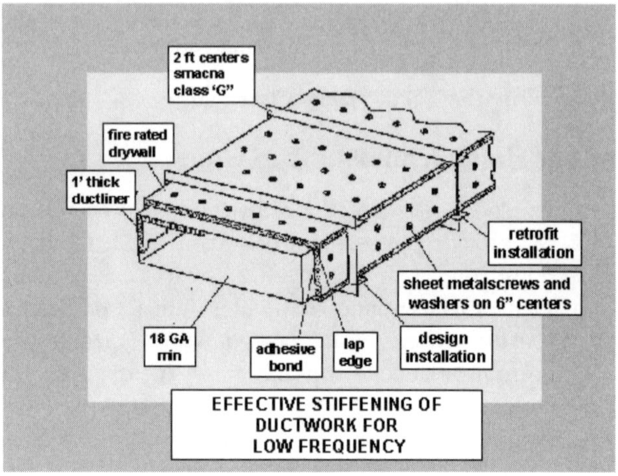

FIGURE 6-3 Increasing the stiffness of discharge ductwork by attaching drywall.

occupied space. Alternately use carefully selected sound attenuators.

3. Allow low-frequency noise to radiate out of the initial part of the supply ductwork by locating the unit over noncritical spaces, such as bathrooms, or by using a side-supply unit.
4. Rooftop units with a side-supply ductwork layout usually transmit a much lower level of rumble noise than downward discharging units because much of the low-frequency energy can radiate out of the side-supply ductwork above the roof where it is not a problem.
5. Provide solid drywall ceiling under first 20 - 30 ft (6 - 9 m) of supply ductwork beyond the point of roof penetration.
6. Packaged silencers may work well for frequencies at 125 Hz and above but can do little to attenuate noise in the critical low-frequency rumble region below 125 Hz (Ebbing and Blazier 1993).

Return noise path noise control

1. Line inlet ductwork with 1 in. (25 mm) thick duct liner from fan inlet to the first noise-sensitive occupied space to reduce noise reaching occupied spaces via the return air connection to the rooftop unit. Alternately use carefully selected sound attenuators.

2. Size inlet ductwork for 1000 fpm maximum velocity.
3. Additional attenuation can be obtained by using one or more bends in inlet ductwork.
4. Use small multiple return air openings in different spaces to take advantage of the significant end reflection losses in the 63 Hz and 125 Hz octave bands, taken as 10 dB in the 63 Hz octave band, as shown in Figure 6-4. These smaller duct openings radiate significantly less low-frequency noise than a one large area return duct opening.

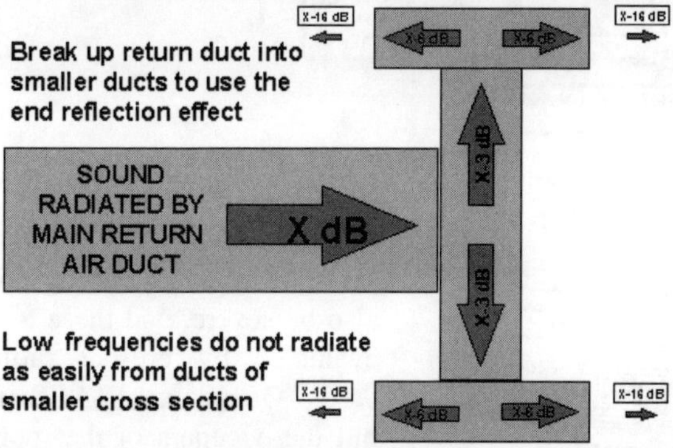

FIGURE 6-4 Attenuation of low-frequency noise from return air ductwork using branching and end reflection effects. This example is for an exit duct with a cross-sectional area less than 2 ft^2.

Rooftop curb to occupied space noise control suggestions

Make sure that the area within the curb that is not used by the supply and return ductwork is filled in with materials that will make the effective sound transmission loss of this part of the roof better than or equal to the rest of the roof. Figure 6-5 shows a suggested treatment. Use a nonhardening, fire-rated caulking and drywall to seal the space between the duct and the roof.

Special Considerations for Packaged Terminal Air Conditioners

The interior bulkhead in a PTAC unit can be critical in controlling the low-frequency transmission of exterior noise to the interior of the building through the wall of the PTAC unit. ASTM E90 STC ratings of the PTAC bulkhead barrier can be misleading because they do not assess low-frequency performance. Compres-

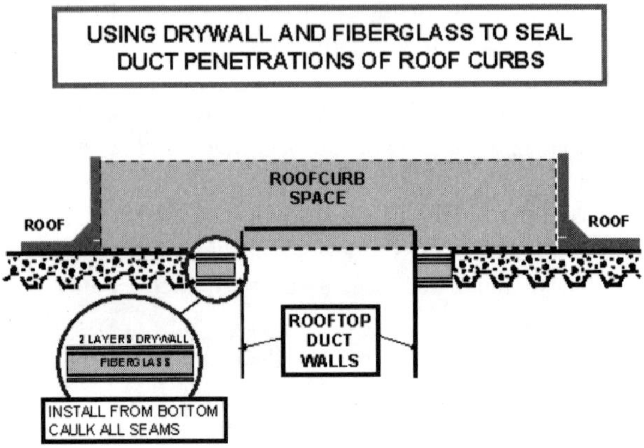

FIGURE 6-5 Recommended curb treatment to attenuate exterior rooftop noise.

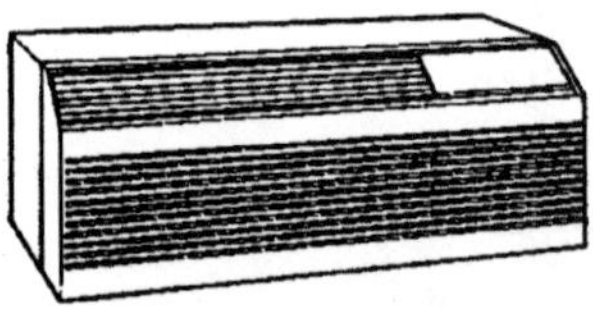

sor starting and stopping noises can also be severe, and these too are not evaluated by present rating standards. Oversizing PTACS may permit the occupant of the room to run the unit at a lower fan-speed setting for reducing indoor fan noise, but this can cause short-cycling of the compressor, which may increase annoyance.

Special Considerations for Water-Source Heat Pumps

The noise sources in WSHPs are the compressor(s), fans, and circulating water pump. The compressors may be reciprocating, rotary, or scroll type. Each of these compressors has different acoustical characteristics. The smaller units usually have single compressors. Higher capacity WSHPs may use multiple compressors, providing for capacity modulation.

INDOOR AIR SYSTEM

Console WSHP models are designed for free delivery of the conditioned air, while other types of WSHP units have ducting capabilities. Smaller WSHPs have multi-speed, direct-drive centrifugal fan systems. Large capacity equipment has belt-drive systems.

- Compressors, fan motors, and fans can generate pure tone noise and low-frequency noise not evident in either the octave band or the A-weighted bel rating.

- Water-source heat pump compressors are sensitive to water-flow balance conditions, which may be ideal at the manufacturers' test stand but not perfectly balanced in the application.
- Ductwork and water piping connected to units can change the noise output. For example, rigid pipe connections can transmit compressor and motor vibration at 120 Hz tonal components to adjacent metal studs and drywall surfaces.
- All types of units should be inspected after installation to ensure that all noise-producing components are vibration isolated from the frame and cabinet. Ensure that all shipping hold-down bolts have been removed. Make sure that compressor piping does not touch the cabinet housing of the unit. Condensate drains should be connected through flexible hoses.
- Unit filters must be kept clean. Dirty filters cause increased static pressure losses and extra fan noise because of a shift in the point of operation of the fan performance curve.
- WSHP units are inappropriate for mounting in critical noise-sensitive spaces.
- The "grade" of the motor should be checked against the original specifications since some motors are much nosier than others.
- Outlet duct configurations should be configured in a straight runout from the discharge connection to the unit, and duct turns close to the unit discharge should be avoided.
- Do not locate units over return air openings.
- If available, specify multiple-speed motors to allow occupants to reduce fan motor speed as needed.

Special Considerations for Vertical Air Conditioners

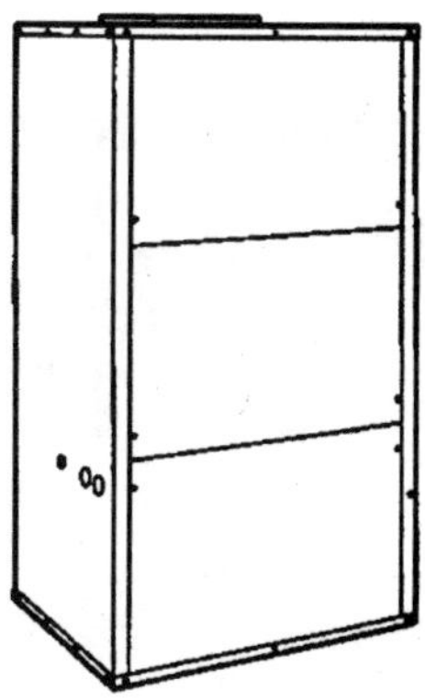

Vertical air conditioners (self-contained units) are often located near occupied spaces. Units of less than 15 tons are often placed inside a closet with a discharge grille penetrating the common wall to the occupied space. Larger units have their own equipment room and duct system. Three common sound paths to consider include:

- fan inlet and compressor sound that radiates through the unit casing to enter the space through separating walls;

- fan discharge sound that is airborne through the supply duct and enters the space through duct breakout and diffusers;
- fan inlet sound finds its way to the space through the return air system.

VIBRATION ISOLATION CONSIDERATIONS FOR PACKAGED PRODUCTS

The adequate vibration isolation of rooftop equipment depends upon the relationship between the static defection of the vibration isolator and the incremental deflection of the supporting roof due to the added weight of the equipment. When the deflection of the supporting roof due to the incremental weight of the unit begins to approach a significant fraction of the isolator static deflection, the ability of the isolator to function as intended is substantially less than that usually indicated in the isolator manufacturer's literature. The performance claims made for vibration isolation by many manufacturers are typically based on an assumption that the supporting structure is infinitely stiff relative to the stiffness of the isolator and, thus, undergoes no deflection of its own. This condition is never approached by roof structures where rooftop units are typically installed.

For example, if the deflection of the roof structure under the load of the equipment is equal to the deflection of the isolator, 50% of the vibratory force is transmitted to the supporting structure. When 10% of the force is to be transmitted, the static deflection of the vibration isolator must be at least eight times greater than the incremental deflection of the floor due to the addition of the equipment load. In the typical lightweight roof structural system, an isolator deflection of several inches is frequently required to effectively vibration-isolate a rooftop unit.

Before installing a rooftop unit, it is always advisable to have a structural analysis made to first determine if the additional deflection in the supporting system is likely due to the equipment load and then to choose an isolator whose static deflection under the weight of the equipment is at least eight times greater.

The popular 1 in. static deflection spring isolator is usually wholly inadequate.

SUGGESTED NOISE AND VIBRATION ISOLATION SPECIFICATIONS

NOISE SPECIFICATIONS

All rooftop units listed in the table below shall have been tested in accordance with ARI Standard 260, Sound Rating of Ducted Air-Moving Equipment. *When operating at the operating points shown, the values of sound power level* (L_W) *shall not exceed those listed in Table 6-6.*

Noise radiated to the outdoors from the units listed in the schedule below shall have been tested in accordance with ARI 270 for units below 10 tons, or ARI 370 for units 10 tons and above. At the operating points listed, the values of sound power level (L_W) *shall not exceed those scheduled in Table 6-6.*

TABLE 6-6
Sample Rooftop Specification

Maximum L_w Values in dB *re* 1 Picowatt Octave Band Center Frequency in Hz											
Mark	cfm	tsp	Source	63	125	250	500	1k	2k	4k	8k
RTU-1	7000	4.5	Discharge								
RTU-1	7000	2.2	Inlet								
RTU-1	---	---	Outdoor								

VIBRATION SPECIFICATIONS

Vibration isolation should be in accordance with Table 42, Chapter 43, *1995 ASHRAE Handbook—Applications.*

REFERENCES

Ebbing, C.E., and W.E. Blazier. 1993. Avoiding low-frequency noise in packaged equipment. *ASHRAE Journal* pp. 46-52, June.

Ebbing, C.E., D. Fragnito, and S. Inglis. 1978. Control of low-frequency duct-generated noise in building air distribution systems. *ASHRAE Transactions* 84(2): 191-203.

Schaffer, M.E. 1991. *A practical guide to noise and vibration control for HVAC systems*, p. 52. Atlanta: American Society of Heating, Refrigerating and Air-Conditioning Engineers, Inc.

SMACNA. 1985. *HVAC duct construction standards—Metal and flexible*, 1st ed. Vienna, Va.: Sheet Metal and Air-Conditioning Contractors' Association.

Chapter 7
Silencers for HVAC Systems

by *Brian Guenther, Tom Paige, and Raymond Vanderburgh*

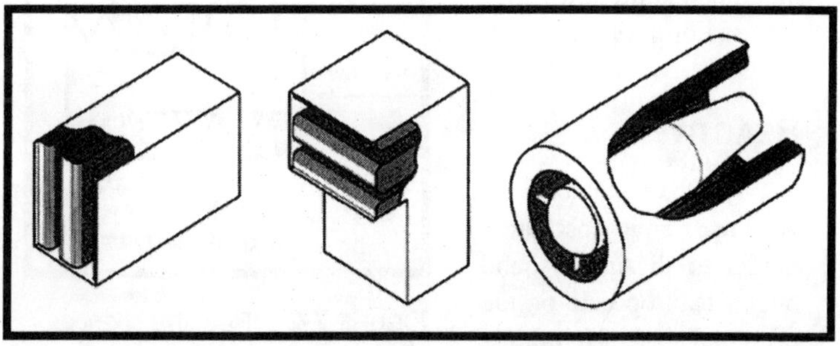

OVERVIEW

Silencers, sometimes referred to as “sound attenuators,” “sound traps,” or “mufflers” are products designed to reduce the airborne noise transmitted from a noise source to a receiver. There are silencers for fans, cooling towers, air-cooled condensers, compressors, gas turbines, and many other pieces of commercial and industrial equipment. For HVAC applications, silencers are normally installed on the intake or the discharge side (or both) of a fan or air-handling system. Also, they may be used on the receiver side of other noise generators such as terminal boxes, valves, and dampers. This chapter is limited to the use of silencers for HVAC applications. General information on these silencers can be found in ASHRAE publications (ASHRAE 1995; Schaffer 1991).

SILENCER TYPES

There are three general types of silencers:

- Dissipative
- Reactive
- Active

Dissipative

Dissipative silencers use absorptive media, such as glass fiber, as the principal sound-absorption mechanism. The glass fiber is protected from the airstream by perforated metal and sometimes with the addition of cloths or films.

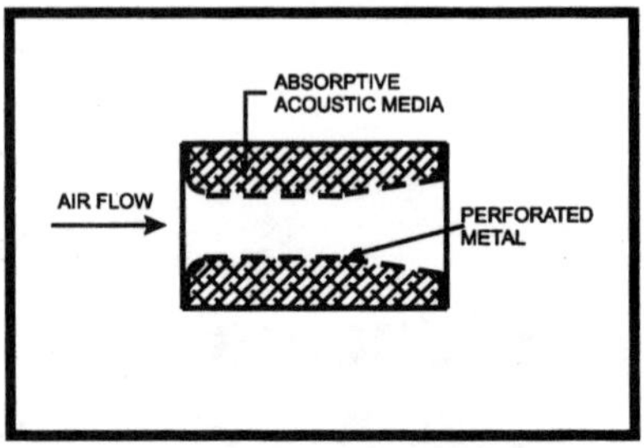

Figure 7-1 Dissipative silencer.

Reactive

Reactive silencers do not use any absorptive media to dissipate sound but instead operate on the principal of Helmholtz resonators. They are constructed only of metal, both solid and perforated. Chambers of specially designed shapes and sizes behind the perforated metal are tuned as resonators or expansion chambers to react with and reduce the sound power at selected frequencies.

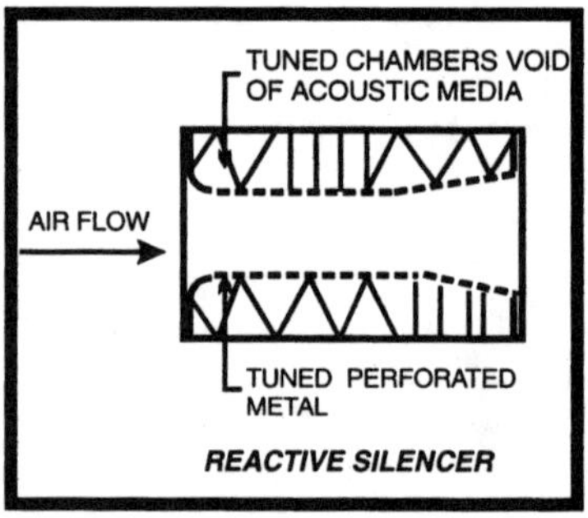

Figure 7-2 Reactive silencer.

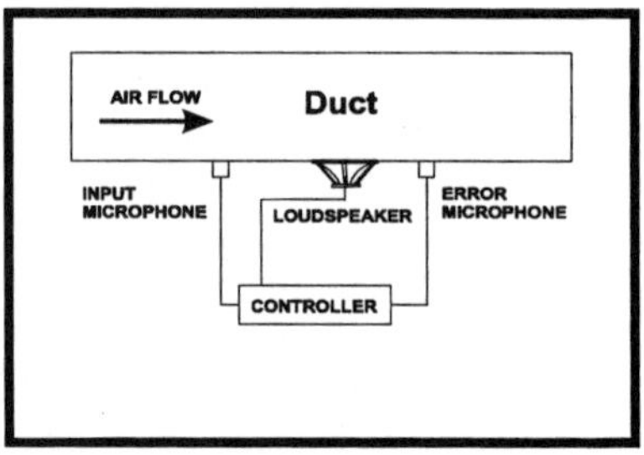

Figure 7-3 Active silencer.

Active

Active silencers, sometimes referred to as "noise canceling systems," electronically generate sound equal in amplitude to the input sound but opposite in phase. The result is the noise transmitted downstream is attenuated by phase cancellation.

RATING TERMINOLOGY FOR SILENCERS

All silencers can be rated for insertion loss, pressure drop, and airflow generated noise.

INSERTION LOSS

Insertion loss (IL) refers to the reduction in sound power level, at a given location, after a silencer is installed ("inserted") in the system. A silencer's insertion loss is measured in decibels as a function of frequency in one-third octave bands and commonly published in full octave bands from 63 Hz to 8000 Hz. The latest revision (ASTM 1996) to the silencer test standard ASTM E-477 contains a significant change in how the full octave-band IL values are computed from the measured one-third octave values. Differences between the revised and previous standards of up to ± 4 dB in the 63,125 Hz and 8000 Hz octave bands may result. Smaller differences may occur in the other octave bands.

Dynamic insertion loss (DIL) is used to identify ratings obtained with airflow present in the system, rather than under static conditions. The DIL rating of a silencer is a function of the air velocity and the direction of flow through the device, relative to that of the sound propagation. "Forward flow" ratings are applicable to silencers installed on the discharge side of fans or "reverse flow" when installed on the fan inlet.

Generally, if dissipative silencers are selected to operate in the proper pressure drop range (0 in. to 0.35 in. or 90 Pa including system effects), the silencer's DIL will not significantly vary from the statically determined IL (usually 1 dB to 2 dB). The effect of airflow on reactive silencers can be much more significant (3 dB to 5 dB).

PRESSURE DROP

Pressure drop (PD) is defined as the differential in measured total pressure across a silencer at a given velocity, usually reported in inches of water or Pascals. A good aerodynamic flow profile is required at both the inlet and discharge of the silencer for accurate measurement. The measuring points usually occur 2.5 to 5 duct diameters upstream and 5 to 10 duct diameters downstream of the silencer in order to avoid turbulent flow areas near the silencer and to allow for any static pressure regain. (A silencer's pressure drop is often mistakenly referred to as "static pressure drop." The static pressure drop may be approximately the same as total pressure drop for silencers located in long uniform ducts. However, static pressure drop is inappropriate when duct expansions or contractions occur within the measurement region.)

Airflow Generated Noise

Airflow generated noise (GN) refers to the sound power generated by the silencer when air flows into, through, and out of a silencer. A silencer's generated noise is measured as a function of frequency (one-third octaves). It is commonly published in full octave bands ranging from 63 Hz to 8000 Hz and is referenced to specific airflow velocities and direction (forward or reverse).

PERFORMANCE CHARACTERISTICS OF SILENCERS

Dissipative Silencers

Dissipative silencer performance is primarily a function of its length; amount of airflow constriction; number, thickness, and shape of splitters or centerbodies; and type, density, and compression of absorptive media. The absorptive media allows dissipative silencers to provide relatively "broad band" (63 Hz to 8000 Hz) insertion loss performance. They are most effective in mid frequencies.

Whenever the absorptive media is faced with a protective lining, such as fiberglass cloth, polyester film, or polyvinyl flouride film, the silencer's insertion loss is usually degraded and generated noise increased (the pressure drop is unaffected). The amount of insertion loss degradation varies with each octave band and thickness and porosity of the lining. It can be as much as 20 dB to 30 dB at certain frequencies. Special methods of applying the protective liner may be used to reduce, but not eliminate, the degradation.

For a given length, silencer designs can produce varying insertion loss and static pressure drop data. Figure 7-4 shows the variation of insertion loss possible for a single manufacturer's line of 5 ft (1500 mm) silencers with pressure drops ranging from 0.10 in. to 0.25 in. at 1000 fpm (25 Pa to 65 Pa at 5 m/s). Even at the same pressure drop, silencers can be configured to provide varying insertion loss performance across the frequency spectrum.

Reactive Silencers

Reactive silencers, in comparison with dissipative silencers,

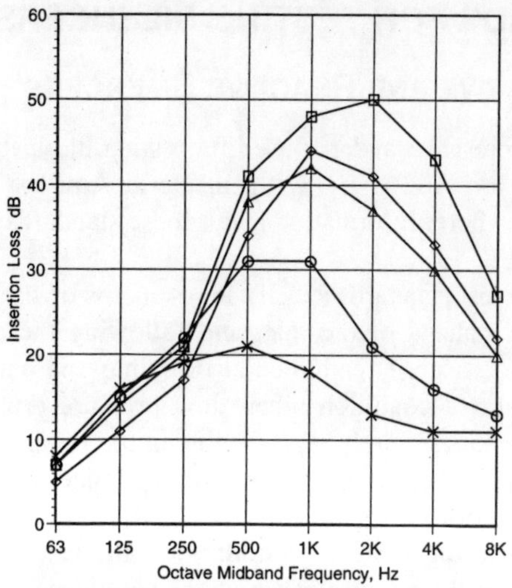

FIGURE 7-4 Insertion loss data for a range of 5 ft (1500 mm) silencers from one manufacturer.

generally have lower insertion loss performance for a given length and pressure drop. Since the insertion loss performance of reactive silencers is largely dictated by the reactive nature of the tuned chambers, the insertion loss spectrum tends to have a sharper peak at certain frequencies. It is more difficult to achieve broad-band insertion loss without absorptive media. Figure 7-5 compares a dissipative silencer's insertion loss (with and without protective lining) against that of a reactive silencer for the same pressure drop.

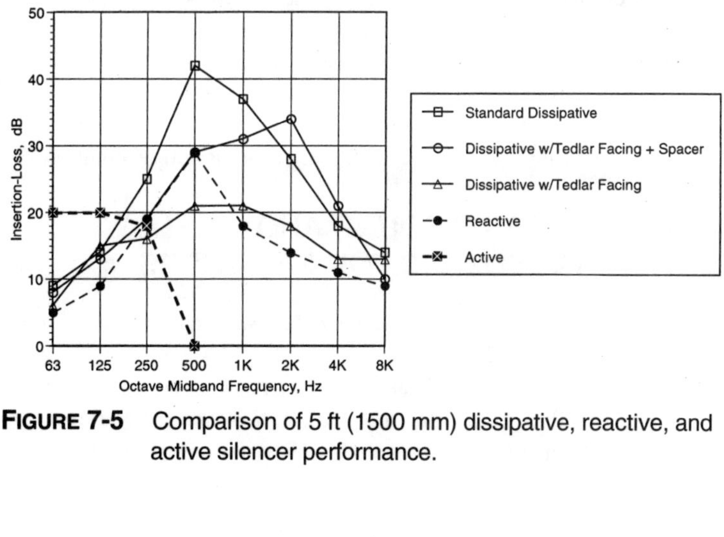

FIGURE 7-5 Comparison of 5 ft (1500 mm) dissipative, reactive, and active silencer performance.

STANDARDS FOR TESTING SILENCERS

DISSIPATIVE AND REACTIVE SILENCERS

The present standards used for testing dissipative and reactive silencers are ASTM E-477-96 in North America and ISO 7235-1991 elsewhere. Information about these standards can be found in Chapter 17.

Both test standards specify long lengths of straight duct (5 dia. to 10 dia.) ahead of the inlet and following the discharge of the silencer to ensure streamlined airflow into and out of the silencer. This creates a condition where low pressure drop values can be achieved that are rarely reproducible in the field. Also, most sound flanking paths are eliminated, which maximizes the silencer's insertion loss performance.

Despite the foregoing similarities, the test standards produce differing results because of variations in loudspeaker (noise source) location/orientation, duct termination conditions, and computation methodology.

In North America, the U.S. Department of Commerce, National Institute of Standards and Technology (NIST) administers the National Voluntary Accreditation Program (NVLAP). Testing laboratories having the proper technical qualifications and competence for conducting the appropriate test methods can be accredited for the ASTM E-477-96 test standard, among others.

ACTIVE SILENCERS

Presently, there are no standard test methods available to test the performance of active silencers. The active silencer's performance greatly depends upon upstream and downstream conditions, duct size, incident noise level and spectrum, etc. Therefore, the user must rely upon the experience and advice of a qualified vendor or consultant when considering the application of active silencers.

MANUFACTURERS' SOUND AND AIRFLOW RATING PROCEDURES FOR SILENCERS

Some manufacturers report dynamic insertion loss data referenced at impractical velocities where pressure drops well exceed 1.0 in. It is important to reference DIL data within the practical pressure drop operating range (0 in. to 0.35 in. or 90 Pa). In this range, the insertion loss variations with airflow will normally be insignificant (less than ± 2 dB).

All testing laboratories have varying sound flanking limitations (usually around 50 dB to 70 dB in the mid frequencies and may be much less at lower frequencies). Reported data for silencers that achieve tested insertion loss values above 50 dB in the mid frequencies are usually truncated at around 50 dB. This recognizes expected flanking limits in the field such as sound traveling down or around the sheet metal walls of the silencer.

As with fans, not all silencers are tested. Some manufacturers' silencer data are derived from interpolation or extrapolation of a set of test data. There is no silencer industry standard similar to AMCA 301 that regulates how the test data are adjusted for untested products. Therefore, it is important to understand how large the manufacturer's test database is and their procedures for interpolating or extrapolating data.

Variations in silencer performance data can occur from manufacturing tolerances. Even carefully crafted production units will vary from a tested unit. Manufacturing deviations in setting internal air passageways can be ±1/8 in. (3.5 mm) or more. This may not

TABLE 7-1
Expected Uncertainties in Silencer Performance Data

Octave Mid-Band Frequency	Measurement Uncertainty of Std. Test Procedure[a]		Expected Reproducibility of Test Data[b]		Production Variability[c]		Random Sample Bias: Catalog vs. Actual[d]	
Hz	IL	GN	IL	GN	IL	GN	IL	GN
63	±1 dB	±2 dB	±3 dB	±10 dB	±1 dB	±3 dB	+3, –8 dB	+15, –5 dB
125-250	±1 dB	±1dB	±2 dB	±6 dB	±1dB	±3 dB	+2, –8 dB	+10, –5 dB
500-4000	±0.5 dB	±1 dB	±1.5 dB	±5 dB	±2 dB	±3 dB	+5, –5 dB	+10, –5 dB
8000	±2 dB	±2 dB	±3 dB	±6 dB	±3 dB	±3 dB	+3, –5 dB	+10, –5 dB
Pressure Drop	±5%		±10%		±10 to 40%		+40%, –5%	

a. Same silencer retested in same lab.
b. Same silencer tested in different labs.
c. Subject to manufacturing tolerances permitted in production quality control.
d. Published catalog data are not customarily derived from a statistical sampling of production units but usually are determined by testing a prototype. Further differences may result from catalog data based on older versions of the test standard.

have much effect on a silencer with a large percentage of open area but could increase the pressure drop of a silencer with a low percentage of open area by an extra 20% to 40+% (Table 7-1). The airflow-generated noise of the same silencer may increase by up to 3 dB or more and the insertion loss may not be significantly affected.

APPLICATION OF SILENCER DATA TO HVAC SYSTEMS DESIGN

Test standards are usually developed to help the user evaluate or compare one product against another under similar conditions. These conditions are usually ideal and not reproducible in the field. Since it is impractical to design a system to emulate a test setup, it is important to learn how to apply test data to actual job installations.

DISSIPATIVE AND REACTIVE

When selecting a silencer, the user should consider the following.

1. How much insertion loss is necessary to achieve the specified room sound criteria.
2. How much additional pressure drop is allowable at the system duct velocity.
3. Where the silencer should be located.
4. How much silencer airflow-generated noise can be tolerated.

Insertion Loss Issues

In determining the insertion loss required, the user should analyze each duct system, summing the noise-generating elements and subtracting the attenuation elements, not including that of the silencer. (See page 43.29, "System Design Procedures," in the *1995 ASHRAE Handbook—HVAC Applications* for more details). The silencer's required insertion loss is the positive difference between the estimated resultant sound pressure level in the space and the room criteria for the space. The user should consider both the supply and return sound paths along the duct to the outlets/inlets as well as potential locations along the system where the sound may break out of the ductwork.

Compare the actual insertion loss spectrum required with the insertion loss spectrum shapes for different silencer sizes and pressure drops available. Select the one that fits the insertion loss required most closely at the pressure drop desired. This will ensure the most energy-efficient selection.

Normally, the selection of a silencer is limited by the space available and allowable pressure drop. It should be recognized that, for a given length, the pressure drop of a silencer will increase as the square of the proportional increase in duct velocity. Thus, the lower the system velocity, the more insertion loss that can be achieved. In higher velocity systems, longer silencer lengths with larger air passageways may be required to maintain acceptable pressure drops and achieve the required insertion loss.

Pressure Drop Issues

Extra system pressure drop forces the fan to a more loaded and more noisy position on the fan curve. Thus, it is important to determine how much silencer pressure drop (including system effects) has been allowed for in the system design. Ordinarily, the silencer pressure drop (including system effects) should not exceed 0.35 in. (90 Pa).

The user should always consider the added losses due to aerodynamic system effects. That is, if the silencer is located where less than ideal conditions at the inlet and/or at the discharge of the silencer exist, then the silencer's effective pressure drop will be increased. (Total silencer PD = silencer PD per ASTM E-477-96 + system effect losses). In some situations, the added system effect losses can exceed the pressure drop of the silencer.

For example, an elbow fitting located immediately following a silencer will prevent the regain of static pressure from the silencer's exit velocity pressure. Furthermore, local velocities within the elbow fitting will be greater than the average duct velocity, which will produce higher overall static pressure losses. (See Figure 7-6).

Some manufacturers give guidelines to estimate increased pressure losses due to varying silencer inlet and discharge conditions (Table 7-2). These should be considered only very approximate

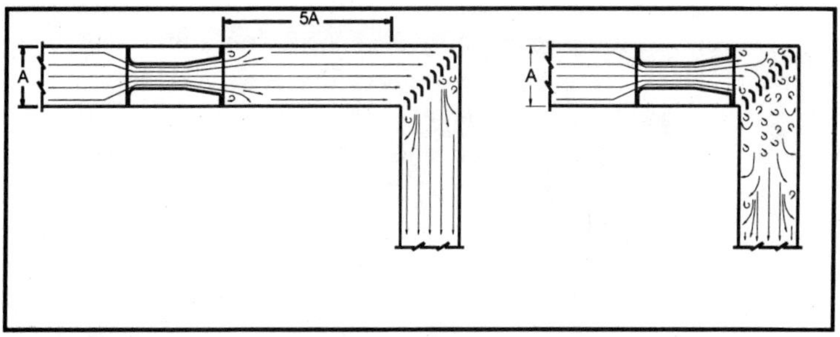

FIGURE 7-6 Effect of silencer location on pressure drop performance.

TABLE 7-2
Some Approximate Silencer System Effect Factors

Silencer Inlet Condition (Within 3-4 Duct Diameters of Silencer Inlet)	Pressure Drop Factor[a]
Straight Unobstructed Duct	1.0
Free Air/Plenum with Smooth Inlet	1.05
Radius Elbow (with Turning Vanes)	1.05
Radius Elbow (No Turning Vanes)	1.1
Miter Elbow	1.30
Free Air/Plenum with Sharp Inlet	1.10 - 1.30
Fan	1.1 - 1.25
Silencer Outlet Condition (Within 5 Duct Diameters of Silencer Outlet)	**Pressure Drop Factor**
Straight Unobstructed Duct	1.0
Duct Doubles Area Abruptly	1.40
Radius Elbow (with Turning Vanes)	1.50
Radius Elbow (No Turning Vanes)	1.90
Miter Elbow	2.0
Abrupt Expansion/Plenum	2.0
Fan	1.20 - 1.40

a. Silencer Pressure Drop (including system effects) = Silencer Pressure Drop per test code × Pressure Drop Factor (inlet) × Pressure Drop Factor (outlet).

guidelines. Substantial variations can occur depending upon the type of silencer, its internal geometry, size of silencer, size of duct, airflow turbulence, etc.

In some situations, transitions can be added to the inlet and outlet of the silencer to increase its cross-sectional area, reduce the airflow velocity, and, thus, reduce the silencer's pressure drop. However, this must be carefully evaluated. Transitions with angles greater than 7.5° can cause turbulence in the silencer, prevent static pressure regain on the discharge, and actually increase the silencer's pressure drop and generated noise. Transitions also lengthen the space required for the silencer.

Transitions may also be required for silencers that are only available in certain limited sizes. However, many manufacturers produce silencers that fit the actual project ductwork and eliminate the need for the added cost and energy consumption of transitions.

SILENCER LOCATION

Silencers should generally be located as close to the fan or noise source as possible. This will help contain the noise at the source and limit potential points along the system where the unsilenced noise may break out. However, turbulent airflow usually exists close to noise sources such as fans, valves, dampers, etc. Therefore, the user should evaluate aerodynamic system effects.

If silencers are carefully designed, they can actually improve flow conditions close to fans. Special fan inlet and discharge silencers, including cone silencers and inlet box silencers, minimize aerodynamic system effects and contain noise at the source. Their effective added pressure drop could be slightly negative if the silencer improves the flow into or out of the fan, thus increasing the fan's performance.

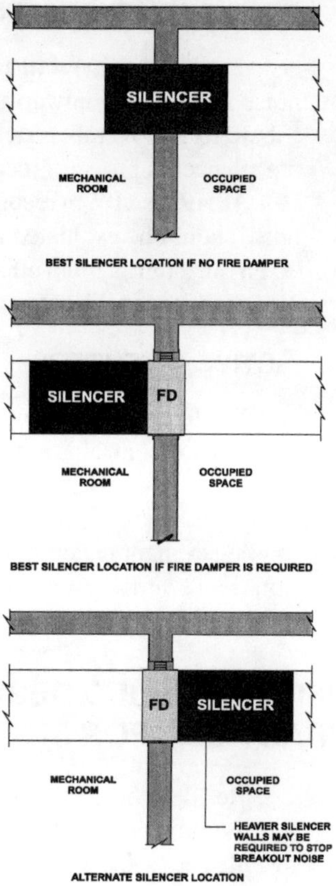

FIGURE 7-7 Considerations for silencer location.

Generally, the best acoustic location for a duct silencer is straddling the mechanical room wall to minimize ductborne and breakout/break-in noise (Figure 7-7). However, fire dampers are usually located at this point. As a compromise, many times silencers are located inside the mechanical room just before the mechanical room wall. If space does not permit, the silencer may need to be located outside of the mechanical room. In this case, heavier silencer walls may be required to prevent noise from breaking out of the silencer before it is fully attenuated.

AIRFLOW-GENERATED NOISE ISSUES

In the majority of installations, a concern for airflow-generated noise is generally unwarranted because it does not materially contribute to the overall system noise level. This is particularly true if the silencer is properly located close to the source.

ASHRAE (1995) recommends that, in general, airflow-generated noise should be evaluated if static pressure drops exceed 0.35 in. or 90 Pa (including system effects), the noise criterion is below RC-35(N), or if the silencer is located very close to or in the occupied space.

ACTIVE SILENCERS

While useful for low-frequency sound (31.5 Hz to 250 Hz), active noise control is not yet a commonly applied silencing product for HVAC systems. Actual noise reduction is system specific. There are no test methods or off-the-shelf data to use. Therefore, it is best to contact manufacturers of these systems for application information. Field verification of manufacturers' data is simply a matter of turning a switch on and off.

RECOMMENDED DESIGN AND INSTALLATION PRACTICES FOR SILENCERS

Besides the location issues discussed above, dissipative and reactive silencers need no special installation instructions if installed by a sheet metal craftsperson. Following are some helpful suggestions.

- Keep duct transitions gradual (less than 7.5° total angle).
- Wherever possible, keep distance between duct fittings (elbows, T's, dampers) and standard straight silencers no closer than three duct diameters; consider elbow silencers when space is limited.
- Wherever possible, keep distance between fans and standard straight silencers no closer than one duct diameter (or hydraulic diameter) for each 1k ft/min (5 m/s) of airflow.
- Match cone silencer "centerbodies" to either the axial fan hub or motor sizes.
- When rectangular silencers are located before or after elbows, keep splitter orientation so that they are in the plane of the elbow.
- In rectangular silencer banks, orient the splitters vertically to help provide structural rigidity.

SUGGESTED SOUND AND AIRFLOW SPECIFICATIONS FOR SILENCERS

Sample Silencer Specification

All silencers listed in the schedule below shall have been tested in a NVLAP accredited laboratory for ASTM E-477-96, Standard Test Method for Measuring Acoustical and Airflow Performance of Duct Liner Materials and Prefabricated Silencers. *The test shall be in strict conformance with ASTM E-477-96 and shall measure insertion loss at appropriate airflow, pressure drop, and noise generation in the same facility. Acoustical data shall be reported in octave bands at center frequencies from 63 Hz to 8 KHz.*

Table 7-3
Sample Silencer Specification

TAG	cfm	Vel.[a] (fpm)	Maximum Pressure Drop (in. w.g.)	Minimum Insertion Loss (dB)							
				63	125	250	500	1k	2k	4k	8k
SL-1	20,000	+733	0.15	8	15	14	14	12	10	9	5
SL-2	15,000	–500	0.10	5	8	15	18	24	23	10	11

a. The symbol "+" designates forward flow and the symbol "–" designates reverse flow.

Insertion losses listed in the table are minimums; pressure drops are the maximum allowable.

Important Considerations When Specifying Silencers

The specified insertion loss should be that calculated to meet the system requirements, not a particular manufacturer's silencer data. It may be impossible for one manufacturer to exactly duplicate another manufacturer's silencer data for all frequency bands. Yet, this same manufacturer may have a product that will meet the actual project requirements.

The silencer's pressure drop should be specified as per ASTM E-477-96 rated values. While the designer must allow for system effect losses, these additional losses should not be included in the specified values. Doing so may result in a silencer manufacturer selecting a silencer with a higher pressure drop than intended.

If system analysis and calculations have been made to determine maximum allowable silencer airflow-generated noise values, then these values, not a particular manufacturer's silencer data, should be specified.

For critical jobs or those with multiple systems, consider specifying mock-up testing. For very critical jobs, consider a witness test of the mock-up(s).

The specification for active silencers needs to be coordinated with the manufacturer.

SUMMARY

Actual field-installed silencer performance will vary from manufacturers' published data due to the following:

- Variations among ASTM, ISO, and other silencer test standards
- Test standard repeatability (silencer re-installed in the same test setup)
- Lab-to-lab reproducibility (same silencer tested in different labs)
- Manufacturers' interpolation and/or extrapolation of test data
- Manufacturing tolerances (actual production unit different than test unit)
- System effects

To minimize uncertainty of the above, carefully performed mock-up testing can provide the closest prediction to actual installed performance. Considering the data variations in other components such as fans and terminal devices, especially at low frequencies (63 Hz and below), mock-up testing can prove to be well worth the investment.

REFERENCES

ASHRAE. 1995. *1995 ASHRAE handbook—HVAC applications*, pp. 43.17, 43.29. Atlanta: American Society of Heating, Refrigerating and Air-Conditioning Engineers, Inc.

ASTM. 1996. *ASTM E-477-96, Standard test method for measuring acoustical and airflow performance of duct liner materials and prefabricated silencers*. Philadelphia: American Society for Testing and Materials.

Schaffer, M.E. 1991. *A practical guide to noise and vibration control for HVAC systems*, pp. 29-32. Atlanta: American Society of Heating, Refrigerating and Air-Conditioning Engineers, Inc.

Chapter 8
Roof Ventilators

by *John A. Paulauskis and Warren Blazier*

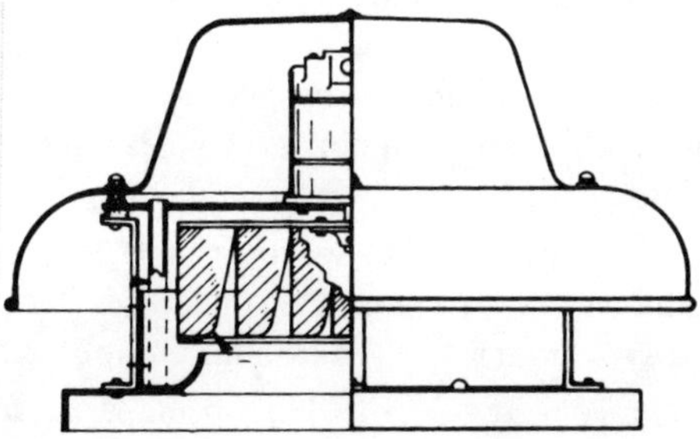

OVERVIEW

Roof ventilators are used in HVAC systems to exhaust air from specific areas such as kitchens, toilets, laboratories, etc. The typical range of fan performance extends from about 100 cfm to 15000 cfm, at static pressures on the order of 0.05 in. w.g. to 3.0 in. w.g. Roof ventilators vary in physical size from about 1 ft to 5 ft in diameter and height. The fan is typically a single-inlet, backwardly inclined centrifugal. Vibration is usually not a problem in the smaller size units (fan diameters less than about 24 in.), but it can become significant in the larger sizes.

MANUFACTURERS' SOUND RATING PROCEDURES AND PRACTICES FOR ROOF VENTILATORS

Octave-Band Sound Power Level

Roof ventilator fan equipment is tested in accordance with AMCA Standard 300. The results are usually expressed in terms of octave-band sound power levels as a function of frequency over the range from 63 Hz to 8000 Hz. This information is valuable to the design engineer because it forms the basis for determining appropriate system noise control measures when acoustical performance is frequency-sensitive. Data obtained using AMCA 300 is available in one-third octave bands from manufacturers. One-third octave-band data are of great value in determining the presence of potentially annoying tonal components, such as the blade-passage frequency (number of blades × rpm/60), that may require attention in the noise control design of the system.

A-Weighted Sound Power Level, $L_W(A)$

In addition to the procedure for determining octave-band sound power level using AMCA Standard 300, AMCA Standard 301 also specifies another procedure for calculating the A-weighted sound power level, $L_w(A)$, of the fan noise. This is a single-number rating that is obtained by weighting the frequency content of the unweighted sound power level spectrum in a manner analogous to the way the human ear perceives the sound.

The $L_w(A)$ is primarily used in outdoor noise situations where many environmental regulations have been expressed in terms of the permissible A-weighted sound pressure level, $L_p(A)$, at some specified distance or location from the source. However, in order to estimate compliance in a given application, source to receiver correction factors for distance and shielding are applied to the $L_w(A)$ rating to convert to $L_p(A)$ (see Chapter 2). Unfortunately, the $L_{w+}(A)$ rating gives no information about the frequency content of the noise spectrum. Therefore, if it is necessary to take remedial noise control measures to comply with a regulation, such as the construction of a shielding barrier, octave-band sound power level data must be obtained from the manufacturer from tests made in accordance with AMCA 300.

Relative Loudness in Sones

Some manufacturers of ventilation fans rate the acoustical performance of their products in sones, using a procedure provided in AMCA Standard 301. A sone rating is a measure of the relative loudness of one sound with respect to another. In practice, the use of sone ratings is almost universally discouraged by knowledgeable engineers and consultants because no meaningful comparison can be made between products in terms of the potential for annoyance as perceived by the listener. For example, it is quite possible for two different fan designs to have identical sone ratings but to be assessed dramatically different on the basis of subjective annoyance (see Chapter 3).

Test Configurations

One of the reasons for the lack of uniformity in the publication of sound data on roof ventilators is the variability of fan configurations. For example, typical configurations are:

- free inlet/free outlet,
- free inlet/ducted outlet,
- ducted inlet/free outlet, and
- ducted inlet/ducted outlet.

Therefore, if acoustical information is to be obtained in accordance with AMCA 300 that separates inlet from discharge noise, eight different setup configurations and eight series of tests are required for each fan. Thus, to reduce cost, manufacturers typically test only a few types and sizes using the laboratory procedures specified by AMCA 300 and then extrapolate the results to calculate the performance of other sizes and types using AMCA 301.

APPLICATION OF ROOF VENTILATOR SOUND RATINGS IN BUILDING SYSTEMS

Uncertainty in Measured Data

One can expect the AMCA-300 octave-band sound power levels provided by manufacturers to have measurement uncertainties generally on the order of the values shown in Table 8-1. These uncertainties reflect not so much a lack of precision in using the AMCA procedure, but the fact that there is variability among manufacturers laboratories due to differences in the physical size, geometry, and acoustical properties of the test facilities, and testing differences that will also occur in the field.

System Effects

Roof ventilators are generally installed on roof curbs, as shown in Figure 8-1. Within the curb space, backdraft dampers are installed to prevent outside air from entering the building when the fan is not operating. This damper not only adds pressure drop to the fan system (not included in the laboratory rating) but also creates

TABLE 8-1
Estimated Variability of Product Sound Power Data Due to Measurement Uncertainties and Production Quality Control
The Frequency Bands Most Affected by System Effects in the Application are Also Indicated in the Shaded Areas.

Roof Ventilators						
Octave Mid-Band Frequency Hz	Measurement Uncertainty of Std. Test Procedure[a] dB	Repeatability of Test Data[b] dB	Production Variability[c] dB	Cumulative Uncer-tainty Due To All Previous Factors[d] dB	Variability of Random Sample *re* Catalog[e] dB	Bands Most Affected by System Effects[f] dB
63	± 4 dB	± 2 dB	± 4 dB	± 6 dB	+6, -0	+5 to15 dB
125	± 3 dB	± 1 dB	± 3 dB	± 4 dB	+5, -0	+5 to15 dB
250	± 2 dB	± 1 dB	± 3 dB	± 4 dB	+3, -0	+5 to15 dB
500-4000	± 1.5 dB	± 1 dB	± 3 dB	± 4 dB	+3, -0	+0 to 5 dB
8000	± 3 dB	± 0.5 dB	± 3 dB	± 4 dB	+3, -0	+0 to 5 dB

a. Standard deviation of octave-band data per ISO 3741.
b. Repetitive testing of same unit in same laboratory.
c. Subject to manufacturing tolerances permitted in production quality control.
d. Based on the square root of the sum of the squares of all uncertainties.
e. Published catalog data are not customarily derived from a statistical sampling of production units but usually are determined by testing a prototype. Thus, the results of testing random production samples would tend to exceed those published by the manufacturer.
f. See below for a discussion of application-related system effects.

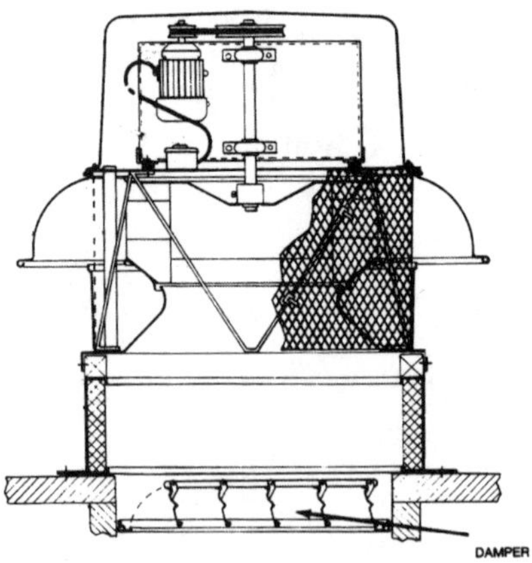

FIGURE 8-1 Roof ventilator installation.

additional air turbulence at the fan venturi, thereby introducing a system effect with increased fan noise. Frequently, poor installation or weathering of the damper will cause it to bind in less than a full open position, creating even more air turbulence and a greater system effect (see Figure 8-2a). The additional pressure drop created by the backdraft damper often results in reduced airflow, which forces an increase of the fan speed at the time of commissioning. Increased fan speed will increase fan noise above the manufacturers' rating in most of the frequency bands by an amount equal to 50 log (RPM_F / RPM_I) dB, where RPM_F = final fan speed, and RPM_I = initial fan speed. For example, a 20% increase in speed results in a 4 dB increase in noise level. Nonvaned duct elbows are frequently located directly below power roof ventilator inlets. This creates nonuniform airflow at the inlet venturi to the fan and introduces excessive air turbulence and swirl, as illustrated in Figure 8-2b. If the swirl rotation is opposite to the fan rotation, counter-rotating airflow will enter the fan wheel as shown in Figure 8-2c. In the 63 Hz and 125 Hz octave bands, any of these conditions result in at least a 3 dB to 5 dB increase in noise level above the manufacturer's rating.

An often unexpected system effect occurs as a result of installing roof ventilators on sound curbs as a noise control measure. For example, a horizontal baffle type sound curb can generate extra air turbulence at the inlet venturi, as shown in Figure 8-3a. This may cause an increase in noise of up to 5 dB in the 31.5 Hz, 63 Hz, and 125 Hz octave bands. Vertical baffle type sound curbs can also create poor entering flow conditions, as illustrated in Figure 8-3b. Vertical baffles in conjunction with an inlet elbow (Figure 8-3c) can trap air against one side of the sound curb causing a significant pressure drop and increased air turbulence.

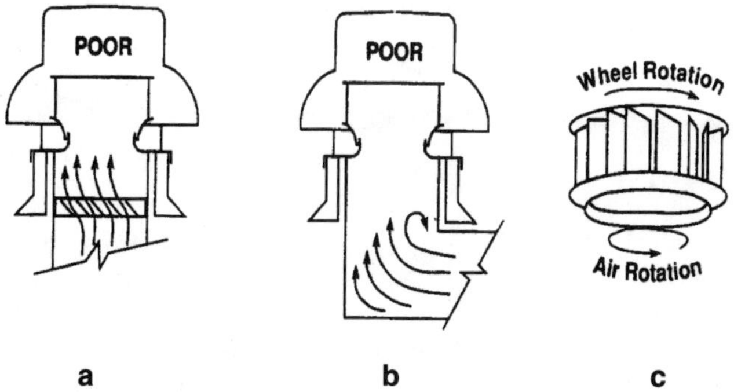

FIGURE 8-2 Inlet conditions on roof ventilators.

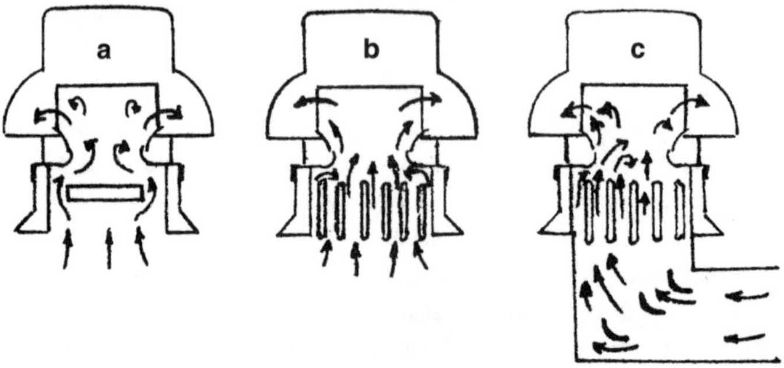

FIGURE 8-3 Sound curb configurations.

As a result of these unanticipated system effects, the installer is usually forced to increase the fan speed to compensate for the loss in air delivery. Because of the substantial increase in fan noise that accompanies the increased fan speed, the noise reduction, which the sound curb was originally designed to provide, may be totally inadequate. Furthermore, the combination of an inlet backdraft damper, elbow, and sound curb can often introduce a sufficient increase in the static pressure requirement as to necessitate a complete replacement of the unit with one of a larger size.

RECOMMENDED DESIGN AND INSTALLATION PRACTICES FOR ROOF VENTILATORS

LOCATION

When possible, roof ventilators sized for 1500 cfm or greater should not be located directly above noise sensitive space such as conference rooms, private offices, etc. Smaller roof ventilators may be located above such spaces only when adequate noise controls are incorporated into the design. Large roof ventilators exceeding 5000 cfm should always be located above unoccupied spaces such as duct chases, storage rooms, or mechanical rooms.

DESIGN

The lowest possible sound level for a specific type of roof ventilator, at a given airflow and pressure, will usually be achieved when the most efficient fan is selected (i.e., lowest brake horsepower). When requested, manufacturers may be able to provide octave or one-third octave-band sound power level data so that a comparison can be made among several fan selections. A difference in any octave band of 3 dB or less, among fans of similar capacity, is usually not significant in a typical field application.

Design of the inlet duct configuration at a roof ventilator is critical to both the fan noise and airflow performance. The airflow entering the roof ventilator venturi should have a uniform velocity profile and minimum air turbulence without counter-rotation from inlet elbows. Backdraft dampers should be located as far from the inlet venturi as possible and may not even be required for exhaust systems that operate continuously.

Ductwork with ductliner should be substituted for sound curbs to attenuate fan noise whenever possible. Where ductliner is prohibited, as in kitchen and laboratory exhaust systems, efficient fan selection is critical, and the natural noise attenuation resulting from additional unlined duct elbows and longer duct runs should be considered for fan noise control.

VIBRATION ISOLATION

Roof ventilators under 5000 cfm usually do not require vibration isolation. Spring-type vibration isolation may be required for roof ventilators exceeding 5000 cfm when they are installed on metal roofs and above noise-sensitive spaces. One inch static deflection spring isolators, incorporated as part of a curb-mounted isolation base with a neoprene weather seal, are usually sufficient in the installation of larger roof ventilators.

SUGGESTED NOISE SPECIFICATIONS

The procedure described in Chapter 43 of the *1995 ASHRAE Handbook—Applications* can be used by the engineer to estimate the maximum permissible octave-band sound power levels of roof ventilator units in the development of specifications. A suggested form of specification is as follows:

All roof ventilator units listed in the schedule below shall have the AMCA sound seal per AMCA Standard 311 and shall have been tested in accordance with AMCA Standard 300 or latest revision (see Chapter 17). When operating at the scheduled performance, the values of sound power level, L_w, shall not exceed those scheduled in Table 8-2. Submitted data shall include the fan orientation and inlet/outlet orientation according to AMCA Standard 301.

TABLE 8-2
Sample Power Roof Ventilator Specifications

	Maximum Sound Power Level dB Octave Band Center Frequency in Hz									
Mark	**63**	**125**	**250**	**500**	**1k**	**2k**	**4k**	**8k**	**cfm**	**tsp**
RV-1										
RV-2										

Chapter 9
Panel-Type Propeller Exhaust Fans

by *John A. Paulauskis and Warren Blazier*

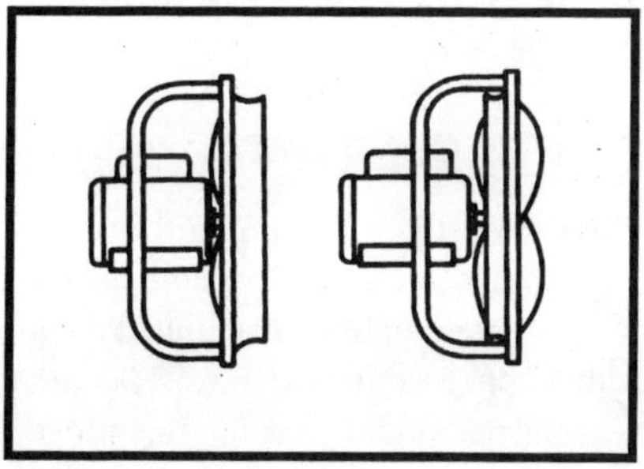

OVERVIEW

Propeller-type exhaust and makeup air fans are similar to inline axial fans, except that they are not ducted. These fans are designed for low pressure applications, and, as such, the pressure rise across the fans is usually limited to 1 in. w.g. or less. Panel-type exhaust fans used in commercial applications are similar to residential window fans except that they are much larger in size and have a variety of alternative blade designs. Large volumes of air are attainable from a single fan (up to 80,000 cfm is typical). Neglecting accessory attachments at inlets and outlets, propeller fans are relatively uniform in overall construction among manufacturers. However, the blade designs vary greatly. Both direct and belt drives are used.

NOISE CHARACTERISTICS OF PANEL-TYPE PROPELLER FANS

There is significant variation among manufacturers in the physical design of panel-type propeller fan equipment. For this reason, there is also a large variation to be expected in fan noise levels among competitive products of similar capacity. These variables in propeller fan design include the blade shape and number, the blade pitch, the fan diameter, and the operating speed. Each of these variables has a significant influence on the noise level produced in a given application. For example, the broad-band noise level of a given fan design increases approximately as the cube of the blade-pitch and the fifth power of the tip speed. In addition to the broad-band noise, a prominent tonal component corresponding to the blade-passage frequency (number of blades × rpm/60) is nearly always present.

MANUFACTURERS' SOUND RATING PROCEDURES AND PRACTICES

AVAILABILITY OF SOUND DATA

At the present time, there is little uniformity in the format manufacturers use to publish acoustical data on panel-mounted propeller fans. Some manufacturers publish calculated data based on generalized equations that appeared in ASHRAE Handbooks prior to 1995; ASHRAE no longer recommends using this procedure. Others publish test data based on *AMCA Standard 300, Reverberant Room Method for Sound Testing of Fans*. Still others provide extrapolated data based on test results on fans of a similar design, following procedures specified in *AMCA Standard 301, Methods for Calculating Fan Sound Ratings from Laboratory Test Data.*

FORMATS OF MANUFACTURERS' SOUND DATA

Octave-Band Sound Power Level

Tests on fan equipment following the procedures specified by AMCA Standard 300 yield data usually expressed in terms of octave-band sound power level as a function of frequency over the range from 63 Hz to 8000 Hz. Such information is of value to the design engineer because it forms the basis for determining appropriate system noise control measures whose acoustical performance is frequency-sensitive. Data obtained using AMCA 300 is available in one-third octave bands from some manufacturers. One-third octave-band data are of great value in determining the presence of potentially annoying tonal components, such as the blade-passage frequency, that may require attention in the noise control design of the system.

A-Weighted Sound Power Level, $L_W(A)$

In addition to a procedure for extrapolation of test data obtained using AMCA Standard 300, AMCA Standard 301 also specifies another procedure for calculating $L_w(A)$ of the fan noise. This is a single-number rating that is obtained by weighting the frequency content of the spectrum in a manner analogous to that of the human ear.

The primary application for this particular rating is in outdoor noise situations where many environmental regulations have been expressed in terms of the permissible A-weighted sound pressure level (dBA) at some specified distance or location. However, in order to estimate compliance in a given application, source-to-receiver correction factors for distance and shielding must be applied to the $L_w(A)$ power level rating to convert to A-weighted sound pressure level. (See Chapter 2 for a discussion of applicable procedures.)

Relative Loudness in Sones

Some manufacturers of panel-type propeller fans rate the acoustical performance of their products in sones, using a procedure provided in AMCA Standard 301. A sone rating is a measure of the relative loudness of one sound with respect to another. In practice, the use of sone ratings is almost universally discouraged by knowledgeable engineers and consultants because no meaningful comparison can be made between products in terms of the potential for annoyance as perceived by the listener. For example, it is quite possible for two different fan designs to have identical sone ratings but to be assessed dramatically differently on the basis of subjective annoyance. (See Chapter 3 for an amplified discussion.)

UNCERTAINTIES IN APPLICATION OF SOUND RATINGS TO BUILDING SYSTEMS

Following the AMCA-300 test procedure, the octave-band sound power levels provided by manufacturers have measurement uncertainties generally on the order of the values listed in Table 9-1. These uncertainties reflect not so much a lack of precision in using the AMCA procedure as the fact that there is variability among manufacturers' laboratories because of differences in the physical size and geometry of the test facilities.

TABLE 9-1
Estimated Variability of Product Sound Power Data Due to Measurement Uncertainties and Production Quality Control
The Bands Most Affected by System Effects and Point of Fan Operation are Also Indicated (Shaded Areas).

Panel-Type Propeller Fans						
Octave Mid-Band Frequency	Measurement Uncertainty of Std. Test Procedure[a] dB	Repeatability of Test Data[b] dB	Production Variability[c] dB	Cumulative Uncer-tainty Due To All Previous Factors[d] dB	Variability of Random Sample *re* Catalog[e] dB	Bands Most Affected by System Effects and Point of Fan Operation[f] dB
31.5	Data not available	Data not available	Data not available	Data not available	Data not available	+5 to15 dB
63	± 4 dB[g]	± 2 dB	± 4 dB	± 6 dB	+6, -0	+5 to15 dB
125	± 3 dB	± 1 dB	± 3 dB	± 4 dB	+5, -0	+5 to15 dB
250	± 2 dB	± 1 dB	± 3 dB	± 4 dB	+3, -0	+0 to 5 dB
500-4000	± 1.5 dB	± 1 dB	± 3 dB	± 4 dB	+3, -0	+0 to 5 dB
8000	± 3 dB	± 0.5 dB	± 3 dB	± 4 dB	+3, -0	+0 to 5 dB

a. Standard deviation of octave-band data per ISO 3741.
b. Repetitive testing of same unit in same laboratory.
c. Subject to manufacturing tolerances permitted in production quality control.
d. Based on the square root of the sum of the squares of all uncertainties.
e. Published catalog data are not customarily derived from a statistical sampling of production units but usually are determined by testing a prototype. Thus, the results of testing random production samples would tend to exceed those published by the manufacturer.
f. See Chapter 1 for a discussion of the effects of system effects on installed noise levels.
g. Based on estimated uncertainties per ARI 280.

SUGGESTED NOISE SPECIFICATIONS

ESTIMATE THE MAXIMUM ALLOWABLE SOUND POWER

By using the acoustic calculation procedure outlined in Chapter 43 of the *ASHRAE Handbook*, the designer can estimate and specify the maximum allowable sound power of central-station air-handling units in each octave band.

NOISE SPECIFICATIONS

A good sound specification requires that the user be provided with the best available sound power level data. Although manufacturers' data are not infallible, they are the best commercially available, provided that all the requirements of the referenced AMCA test standards have been met. The essentials of a good sound specification should include the following:

1. A requirement for the AMCA sound seal on all fans in accordance with AMCA Standard 311.
2. Fans must be tested in accordance with AMCA Standard 300 or the latest revision.
3. Base or extrapolated data must include information on the fan orientation and inlet/outlet conditions according to AMCA 301.
4. Submitted sound power level data should be provided in one-third or full octave bands.
5. Maximum allowable sound power levels (See Table 9-2).

Submit for approval manufacturers' independently certified sound power levels for the eight octave midband frequencies from 63 Hz to 8000 Hz. All fans shall bear the AMCA Sound Seal and shall have been tested in full compliance with AMCA Standards 300, 301, and 311. Submit all fan test setup data required under AMCA Standard 301. Maximum allowable sound power levels for EX-1, EX-2, etc., are specified in Table 9-2.

TABLE 9-2
Sample Panel-Type Propeller Exhaust Fan Specifications

	Maximum Sound Power Level, dB Octave Band Center Frequency in Hz							
Mark	**63**	**125**	**250**	**500**	**1k**	**2k**	**4k**	**8k**
EX-1								
EX-2								

Chapter 10
Grilles, Registers, and Diffusers

by *Ted Carnes and Warren Blazier*

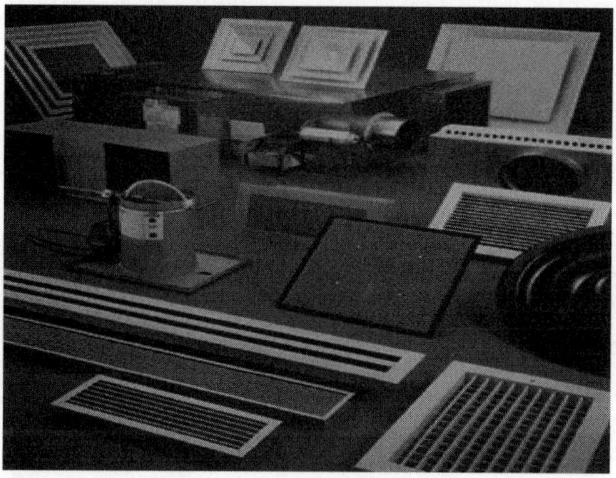

OVERVIEW

Grilles, registers, and diffusers (GRD) are the termination of an HVAC system. These devices are among the most important sources of noise in an HVAC system because they are located within conditioned spaces and are usually in close proximity to the occupants. Grilles, registers, and diffusers can be classified as follows.

- A diffuser is typically mounted flush with a room ceiling and supplies conditioned air that entrains and mixes with room air to temper the thermal environment in the surrounding space.
- A grille is typically mounted in a sidewall and discharges air into the space with some means of deflection control but with

less mixing than obtained with diffusers. A grille may also collect air from the space (a return).

- A register is a grille with an integral flow balancing damper.

In general, diffusers and grilles will contribute something to the sound level in the receiver environment because of "regenerated" noise due to air turbulence created by elements of the interior design, which control the air discharge pattern and optimize the entrainment and mixing of room air. The magnitude of this contribution depends upon the geometry of the design, the uniformity of the inlet air profile, and the volume flow rate. As a rule, there is a direct relationship between diffuser-generated noise and the effectiveness of air distribution: noisy diffusers usually result in better air mixing than quiet ones. Thus, a compromise is generally required between the magnitude of diffuser-generated noise and the quality of air mixing.

In addition, grilles, registers, and diffusers serve as a conduit between the air distribution system and the room by transmitting noise already present in the connected ductwork. For this reason, when sound rating these elements of the duct system it is necessary to utilize a source of "quiet" air to avoid penalizing the device for noise unrelated to the product.

ACOUSTICAL CHARACTERISTICS

Typical GRDs generate noise principally in the octave midband frequency range between 500 Hz and 4000 Hz. This range also corresponds to the major portion of the frequency region associated with human speech. Thus, GRD-generated noise can degrade the quality of speech communication by "masking" if permitted to exceed a certain threshold depending upon the vocal effort used by the speakers (normal vs. raised speaking voice, shouting, etc.).

On the other hand, this speech-masking effect sometimes can be beneficial in open-plan office layouts where a certain degree of conversational privacy between speakers is usually desirable. However, it must be emphasized that GRD-generated noise should only be used for this purpose in constant-volume air distribution systems, where the masking sound can be maintained at a constant, predetermined level. It should not be counted upon in variable-air-volume system applications because the level of GRD-generated noise varies as approximately the fifth power of the flow volume, and, thus, the speech masking capability rapidly diminishes as flow volume is reduced.

MANUFACTURERS' SOUND TESTING, RATING PROCEDURES, AND PRACTICES

Sound Test Procedure

At present, grilles and diffusers are customarily sound tested in accordance with *ASHRAE Standard 70-1991, Method of Testing for Rating the Performance of Air Outlets and Inlets*. This standard covers both aerodynamic and acoustical measurements. ASHRAE Standard 70-1991 references *ANSI S12.31-80, Precision Methods for the Determination of Sound Power Levels of Broadband Noise Sources in Reverberant Rooms*, for acoustical measurements, using the reference-source comparison method. (See Chapter 17 for a description of the substitution/comparison method for determining sound power level.) ASHRAE Standard 70-1991 also specifies the mounting configuration and installation setup for testing the various types of products covered by the standard. Typically, data is obtained at the octave midband frequencies from 125 Hz through 8000 Hz.

However, a significant observation of the procedure is that the specified air supply to the test unit is from a long, straight run of duct that ensures a uniform inlet velocity profile, which is seldom duplicated in a typical field installation of the product. Thus, the test configuration excludes any inlet system effects, and the laboratory test data usually reflect a quieter acoustical performance than will be found in a field application where the inlet supply duct may be close-coupled and frequently offset from the centerline of the unit.

Sound Rating Procedures and Certification

There is presently no recognized industry procedure for sound rating grilles, registers, and diffusers. (The earlier Air Diffusion Council [ADC] 1062 series of testing/rating standards and companion certification program have been inactive since 1985 and should not be referenced in specifications.)

The cognizant trade association is now the Air-Conditioning and Refrigeration Institute (ARI). This organization is currently developing a new rating program based on *ARI Standard 890-94, Rating of Air Diffusers and Air Diffuser Assemblies*, but it has not been implemented at time of publication. ARI Standard 890 references ASHRAE Standard 70 as the method of testing.

Present Manufacturers' Sound Rating Practices: the 10 dB "Room Factor"

Raw test data on the acoustical performance of a GRD device is typically expressed in terms of octave-band sound power levels. Thus, it is necessary to convert the data to sound pressure levels before comparison to a particular noise criterion specified for the application in question. (See Chapter 2 for a discussion of the relationship between sound power level and sound pressure level.)

An appropriate conversion from sound power to sound pressure requires knowledge of the acoustical properties of the receiving space, including the room size and acoustical absorption present, the number of diffusers serving the space, and the distance from the source(s) to the specified receiver location. Because these factors are highly variable from application to application, in order to simplify the publication of cataloged sound rating data, most manufactures assume a "default" value for the conversion factor. Presently, most manufacturers have adopted a default value of 10 dB, independent of frequency, which they then use to calculate a diffuser NC rating (see Chapter 3). However, the use of this 10 dB "room factor" can lead to prediction errors in an application because it does not adequately take into account the effects of room size and the number of diffusers serving the receiving room space.

For example, if a single diffuser serves the receiving room, a conversion factor of 10 dB between source sound power level and room sound pressure level would be appropriate for a room with a 9 ft ceiling height and floor area of approximately 550 ft^2, based on ASHRAE-sponsored research by Schultz (1985). However, this corresponding room size (22 ft × 25 ft) is larger than most private office applications for a single diffuser, and the use of a 10 dB conversion factor in many instances may result in an underprediction of room sound level by several NC points. Table 10-1 lists appropriate values of the conversion factor for private office applications as a function of room size.[1] (Note that in cases where two diffusers might be used to serve a private office as large as 300 ft^2, the conversion factor used for diffuser selection is 3 dB less than if a single diffuser is used. This occurs because each diffuser contributes one-half the permissible total sound power delivered to the receiving space.)

1. Conversion factors for the 500 Hz and 1000 Hz octave bands are illustrated because it is in this frequency region that the NC rating of a GRD noise spectrum will usually be determined for most diffuser types.

TABLE 10-1
Conversion Factor for Private Offices with a 9 ft Ceiling Height

Approximate Room Size	Number of Diffusers	L_w - L_p @ 500 Hz (dB)	L_w - L_p @ 1000 Hz (dB)
125 ft^2	1	6	7
300 ft^2	1	8	9
300 ft^2	2	5	6

Whenever four or more diffusers are used in a distributed ceiling array to serve large areas such as open-plan offices, a modification of the Schultz single-source equation is necessary to take into account the presence of multiple sound sources in a common plane. The appropriate equation applicable to a distributed array of ceiling diffusers may be found in Appendix B, Section B1.7, of ARI Standard 885-90. Table 10-2 illustrates appropriate values of the conversion factor using this equation that corresponds to a room with a 9 ft ceiling height where the variables are the array spacing and floor area served by each diffuser. As in the previous example, values are shown for the 500 Hz and 1000 Hz octave bands because this is the frequency region that usually establishes the value of the NC sound rating typically specified by the user.

TABLE 10-2
Conversion Factor for Open-Plan Offices with a 9 ft Ceiling Height (Four or More Diffusers)

Array Spacing ft	Floor Area/ Diffuser ft^2	L_w - L_p @ 500 Hz	L_w - L_p @ 1000 Hz
10 × 10	100	4	5
12 × 12	150	5	6
15 × 15	250	6	7
20 × 20	400	7	8

Few, if any, manufacturers of GRDs presently publish octave-band sound power level data in their catalogs. Publishing pertinent octave-band data would significantly increase the size of a diffuser catalog, but this may become less of a problem as PC-based electronic catalogs become available. However, such information may be presently available if requested or specified. Most manufacturers' catalog data will continue to be expressed as NC ratings based on a 10 dB conversion factor until an industry standard ultimately is adopted for sound rating GRD products.

BALANCING DAMPERS

Discharge noise from diffusers can be minimized if the supply duct pressure is maintained as low as possible. Balancing dampers, such as those illustrated in Figure 10-1, are used to counter excessive duct pressures but can generate significant noise due to the turbulence created by the pressure reduction necessary to achieve design air volume at the diffuser terminals. This can result in increased noise of 10 NC points, or more, above the normal diffuser NC rating, particularly if the dampers are located in either the diffuser inlet or within 1 to 2 duct diameters upstream and are throttled significantly.

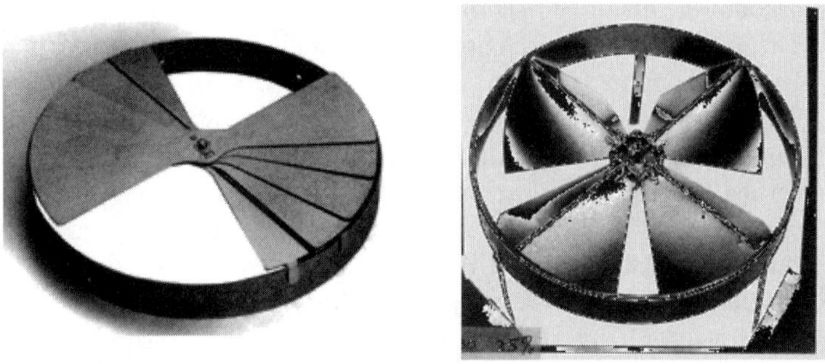

FIGURE 10-1 Typical balancing dampers.

Pressure reducing valves (PRVs) and balancing dampers located at branch take-offs can be effective in achieving design air volume but only if there is sufficient attenuation from lined ductwork installed ahead of the diffuser terminals to attenuate the damper-generated noise.

Even when fully open, these devices can add 5 NC points to a diffusers sound output if located in the diffuser such as for a register. As the balancing damper is closed down, the noise level increase is usually proportional to the cube of the ratio of the diffuser's rated total pressure drop to total pressure in the supply ductwork upstream of the damper. This relationship is illustrated in Table 10-3.

TABLE 10-3
Expected Increase of Close-Coupled Balancing Dampers with Damper Throttling

Ratio of Total Pressure in Duct/ Diffuser Pressure Drop	1	1.5	2	4
Increase in NC points	0	4 - 5	8	16

EFFECT OF NONUNIFORM INLET VELOCITY PROFILE

Ceiling-mounted diffusers, with the limited plenum space available in many installations, can be severely affected by the inlet velocity profile, as illustrated in Figure 10-2. When a flexible connecting duct is offset, or makes a sharp turn at the inlet to a diffuser, both a significant increase in diffuser noise and a poor air distribution profile can result. Where possible, the installation, such as shown in Figure 10-2, should be avoided altogether as the short length of a flexible duct cannot attenuate noise generated by the inlet connection or inlet damper. If the supply duct velocity exceeds 500 fpm, a 45-degree entry or conical tap type connection should be used. (Extractors, which protrude into the main airstream, are not normally recommended but may be considered for special applications.) A minimum of 5 ft of nonmetallic flexible duct should be employed. This will allow smooth radius bends and straight sections before the terminating GRD. See one of the many available references on good duct designs (SMACNA[2] 1993).

For right angle connections, inlet plenums with turning vanes and straightening grids are available and effective (but are seldom specified or installed). Poor inlet conditions can add up to 15 NC points to the rated sound level of a properly selected diffuser. An average effect for a 90° inlet connection is 3 to 5 NC points.

The effect of poor inlet conditions depends partially on the type

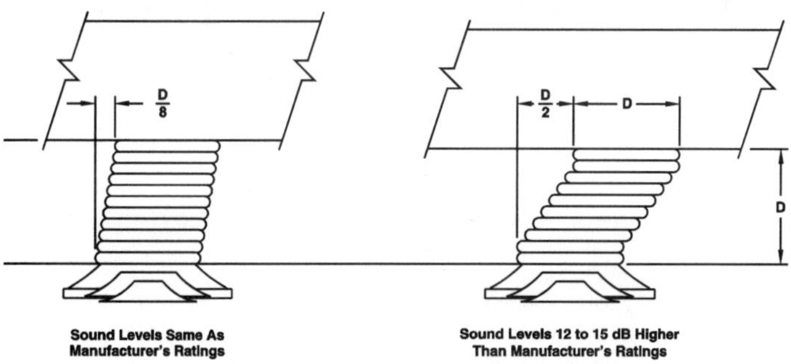

FIGURE 10-2 Effect of entering velocity profile.

2. See SMACNA 1993, Chapter 10, "Provisions for Testing, Adjustment, and Balancing," and Chapter 11, "Noise Control."

of diffuser installed. For example, perforated diffusers with face-mounted deflectors are very sensitive to velocity pattern variations created by inlet flow profiles. Devices with deflectors in the neck are much less sensitive. As a rule, the diffusers with the lowest reported pressure drop for a given flow rate are the most sensitive to inlet flow profiles.

UNCERTAINTIES IN THE APPLICATION OF MANUFACTURERS' DATA

The possible uncertainties in the application of manufacturers' data for grilles, registers, and diffusers are provided in Table 10-4. These are based upon utilized test standards and results found in testing programs.

TABLE 10-4
Estimated Variability of Product Sound Power Data and Bands Most Affected by System Effects[a]

Grilles, Registers, and Diffusers						
Octave Mid-Band Frequency	Measurement Uncertainty of Std. Test Procedure[b] dB	Repeatability of Test Data[c] dB	Production Variability[d] dB	Cumulative Uncer-tainty Due To All Previous Factors[e] dB	Variability of Random Sample *re* Catalog[f] dB	Bands Most Affected by System Effects[g]
63	*	*	*	*	*	*
125	± 3 dB	± 1 dB	± 1 dB	± 3 dB	± 1 dB	
250	± 2 dB	± 1 dB	± 2 dB	± 3 dB	± 2 dB	5 dB
500-4000	± 1.5 dB	± 1 dB	± 2 dB	± 3 dB	± 2 dB	+5 to15 dB
8000	± 3 dB	± 1 dB	± 3 dB	± 4 dB	± 3 dB	

a. Sound power data is seldom available as manufacturers typically list NC values only. For most diffusers, NC is set by sound power in the 500 Hz to 4000 Hz range.
b. Based on ANSI S12-31 for pure tones and assumes that the expected range is 1 standard deviation.
c. Repetitive testing of same unit in same laboratory.
d. Subject to manufacturing tolerances permitted in quality control.
e. Based on the square root of the sum of the squares of all uncertainties.
f. Catalog data for diffusers is based on production samples of common sizes interpolated for all sizes.
g. See discussion of system effects earlier in this chapter.

RECOMMENDED SELECTION AND INSTALLATION PRACTICES

SELECTION

Although an NC 35 criterion is frequently specified as an acoustical design goal in the selection of GRD devices for many building applications, in open-plan office layouts a somewhat higher level of background sound (around NC 40) is occasionally specified to enhance acoustical privacy by masking the intelligibility of conversational speech between occupants outside the local area of the occupant listener.

In fact, the predominant sound produced by typical air diffusers lies within the speech frequency range and is frequently considered as an option to the alternative introduction of masking noise by electronic means.

However, it must be understood that the level and spectrum shape of the masking background sound is relatively critical and only constant-volume air distribution systems can conceivably be used for such an application. If the diffuser sound is too low, the degree of masking is inadequate; if the diffuser sound is too high, or of an inappropriate spectrum shape, the result may be annoying and objected to by the occupant.

The oversizing of diffusers, while providing a quiet installation, often results in a poor air distribution pattern due to the "dumping" of air leaving the diffuser and poor room temperature control. It is far better to reduce the size and capacity of the diffusers and increase their number to obtain an acceptably quiet installation.

INSTALLATION

Duct connections to grilles and diffusers should have no tight bends at the immediate approach to the inlet. (See Figure 10-2 and the discussion above for guidance, along with SMACNA 1993 and manufacturers' installation guidelines and instructions). If balancing dampers are required, they should be located at some distance from the supply outlet, preferably close to a branch take-off, and followed by at least 6 ft of acoustically lined or nonmetallic insulated flexible duct to control the transmission of damper-generated noise.

FLEXIBLE DUCTS

Flexible (flex) ducts provide some "attenuation" of upstream system noise by leaking sound into the surrounding ceiling plenum due to their relatively low wall sound transmission loss and, possibly, their acoustical impedance mismatch effects that would reflect some sound energy back toward the sound source. Because the ceiling beneath the plenum also provides some sound attenuation between the plenum and the room below, the upstream system noise transmitted to the room from the grille or diffuser outlet is reduced. However, flexible ducts, because of their rough interior surface, can also become significant noise generators if flow velocities greater than about 700 fpm are utilized. Thus, in some cases, the attenuation provided by flexible ducts can be offset by the regenerated self-noise if the duct flow velocities are excessive. Flex ducts should not exceed 8 ft in length and should be free of sharp bends.

Vibration Isolation

Grilles, registers, and diffusers are "passive" mechanical devices that require no external vibration isolation. Noticeable vibration and rattling of them are usually a product of excessive air turbulence from upstream of the air outlet devices. Both air outlet and inlet devices are susceptible to structureborne vibration coupled from improperly vibration-isolated rotating mechanical equipment and ductwork or from piping with excessive turbulent flow and mechanical vibration attached rigidly to building structural systems such as the ceiling grid.

Some Practical Noise Control Options

- Reduce the air volume per diffuser by adding additional diffusers. (Down sizing of the diffusers may be necessary if the discharge flow pattern is adversely affected.)
- Install a larger diffuser (oversizing diffusers, however, may reduce air distribution performance).
- Change to a quieter diffuser design.
- Move balancing dampers from the diffuser inlet back to the branch duct take-off point.
- Install rigid rather than flexible duct at the connection to the diffuser and use turning vanes to ensure uniform flow into the diffuser neck. (Be sure that the flexible duct is not, however, required to provide attenuation of upstream noise sources.) If flexible duct is used, keep the inlet to the diffuser free of sharp bends and maintain low inlet velocities.

SUGGESTED ACOUSTICAL SPECIFICATIONS FOR GRDS

Sound data on all GRD devices shall be determined in accordance with ASHRAE Standard 70-1991. The octave-band sound power levels obtained shall be made available upon request. If the manufacturers' simplified catalog data are expressed in NC points, then the magnitude of the acoustical room factor used in the determination of NC shall be stated.

The GRD selection shall be based on the specified NC room criterion adjusted for the difference between the stated assumed room attenuation and that expected at the location of the diffuser, plus expected installation effects.

For example, if the specified room criterion is a NC 35 and the manufacturer has used a 10 dB room factor in cataloging the data, then the following selection guide should be used:

- For a room with 325 ft^2 per diffuser (resulting in a 7 dB room),
- with a typical inlet of flexible duct (which adds approximately 5 NC points),
- select a GRD sound rated at NC 27, as shown below.

NC 35 (Room Requirement):

- 3 NC points (Correction for Room Size) and
- 5 NC points (Inlet Condition Correction).

Results in an NC 27 Maximum Allowable Sound Rating for Selection.

REFERENCES

Schultz, T.J. 1985. Relationship between sound power level and sound pressure level in dwellings and offices. *ASHRAE Transactions* 91(1A): 124-153.

SMACNA. 1993. *HVAC system duct design*, 3d ed. Chantilly, Va: Sheet Metal and Air-Conditioning Contractors' Association.

Chapter 11
Air Terminals

by *Ted Carnes and Warren Blazier*

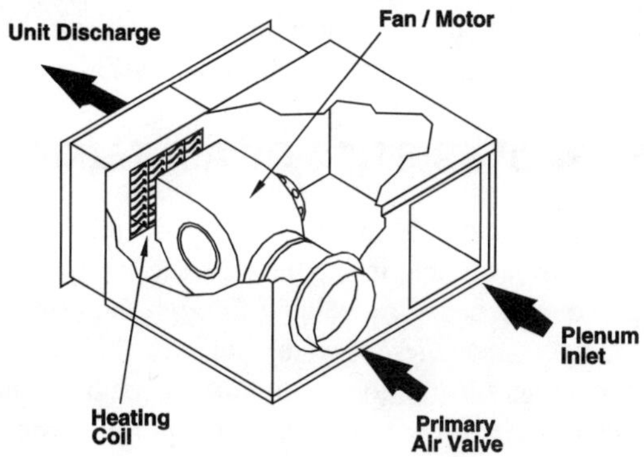

OVERVIEW

Within the context of this chapter, the term *air terminals* refers to a factory-made damper assembly consisting of supply inlet duct connection(s), outlet duct connection(s) or integral air outlets, unit section(s), and fan assembly (when present). Air terminals provide control for individual zones (individual temperature control areas) of conditioned primary air through the use of automatic or manual dampers, valves, heating or cooling coils, nozzles, and fan assemblies.

In general, there are two categories of air terminals: constant air volume (CAV) and variable air volume (VAV). Both types have essentially the same components: a flow rate regulating device (typically a damper, although it may be a bellows or other mechanism) and some method of control. In the simplest of units, the process of controlling the air flow rate generates sound that is proportional to the static pressure drop across the damper mechanism.

In the more complex units that contain induction nozzles or fans, additional sound is generated. Thus, the relationships between the inlet duct static pressure, the primary air flow rate across the damper, and the secondary air flow rate induced by nozzles or an integral fan determine the sound generated by the unit and transmitted to the receiving space.

VAV air terminals are among the most acoustically critical of all HVAC components because they are frequently located directly above occupied spaces. Thus, these units may make a significant contribution to the background sound level in the receiving space, particularly at octave mid-band frequencies from 125 Hz to 2000 Hz. In an RC-type sound analysis (see Chapter 3), the additional sound produced by the air outlets, such as grilles, registers, and diffusers, must also be taken into account. (The acoustical characteristics of these latter components are discussed in Chapter 10.)

NOISE CHARACTERISTICS OF AIR TERMINALS

The basic function of an air terminal device is to reduce the total air pressure available in the inlet duct to the pressure required to deliver the specified flow volume through the downstream system resistance. Since these devices perform this function by the introduction of an obstruction in the airflow path, sound is generated by the aerodynamic turbulence created in the process. In most cases, the sound power level, L_w, produced by the device will be proportional to both the airflow rate and the static pressure drop across the internal damper assembly. In practice, this means that the sound power level, in dB per octave band, is a logarithmic function of the static pressure drop and the flow rate across the damper.[1]

MANUFACTURERS' SOUND RATING PROCEDURES AND PRACTICES FOR AIR TERMINALS

Most manufacturers make data available in two forms for these

1. This can be expressed mathematically as

$$L_w \approx C_0 + K_1 \log(P) + K_2 \log(Q), \text{ dB}$$

where
P = static pressure drop across the unit;
Q = flow rate across the damper;
C_0, K_1, and K_2 are constants determined by test, specific to each octave band and specific to a given unit design.

devices: full octave-band sound power levels at midband frequencies from 125 Hz through 4000 Hz and single-number "Application Data," presented in the form of an NC sound pressure level rating. (Refer to Chapter 3 for a discussion of how NC ratings are obtained.)

The available data is representative of the device only and does not include any external system effects. Data is available over a range of stable operating conditions for both discharge sound (transmitted down the duct) and radiated sound (through either the unit casing or out of the induction port, depending upon the design).

Applicable Acoustical Test and Application Standards

- *ANSI S12.31-1980, Precision Methods for the Determination of Sound Power Levels of Broad-Band Noise Sources in Reverberant Rooms.*
- *ANSI S12.32-1980, Precision Methods for the Determination of Sound Power Levels of Narrow-Band Noise Sources in Reverberant Rooms.*
- *ARI 880-94, Industry Standard for Air Terminals* (and ASHRAE Standard 130P, Method of Testing for Rating of Ducted Air Terminal Units).
- *ARI 885-90, Procedure for Estimating Occupied Space Sound Levels in the Application of Air Terminals and Air Outlets.*

Sound Measurement

Broad-band noise data must be obtained in a reverberant room meeting ANSI Standard S12.31 in order to qualify for testing in accordance with the ARI Standard 880-94 rating requirements. However, if the measurement of narrow-band tonal components is required, such as sometimes produced by fan motors, then the test facility must be qualified in accordance with the ANSI Standard S12.32 procedure.

For most product types, the specified operating point of the test unit for determining the ARI Standard rating is 1.5 in. inlet static pressure at 2000 fpm nominal inlet velocity. Series fan terminals, however, are tested at both maximum rated fan cfm and at reduced fan cfm corresponding to a velocity of 2000 fpm at the primary air inlet.

MEASUREMENT FACILITIES

Ratings based on octave-band sound power levels are determined in a reverberant-room test facility using the reference-source comparison method discussed in Chapter 17. However, a number of manufacturers have also constructed nonstandardized mock-up demonstration facilities for measuring the room sound pressure levels of a unit in a typical field installation. These rooms, which are also used for in situ sound evaluations by listeners, usually have a suspended acoustical ceiling to permit installation in typical plenum configurations and simulate a normal office space. There are no standards covering these types of facilities.

FREQUENCY RANGE OF MEASUREMENTS

The range of normal concern for most air terminal devices is the 125 Hz through 4000 Hz octave mid-band frequencies. The 63 Hz octave band is seldom reported because many manufacturers of these products have reverberation chambers too small to qualify for measurements in this frequency range. However, limited data available from test facilities that can qualify indicates that the level in the 63 Hz octave band is usually less than that in the adjacent 125 Hz octave band. Thus, the absence of 63 Hz octave-band data for these products is not likely to affect the magnitude of the sound rating.

TEST SETUP AND OPERATING CONDITIONS

ARI Standard 880-94 specifies the installation details for sound testing air terminal devices in a reverberant room. Discharge sound power levels are determined by locating the unit outside the test room and connecting it to the reverberant test chamber using a specified length of acoustically lagged 20 ga duct installed flush with the inside wall of the room. The specified length of duct is 2.5 equivalent hydraulic diameters, typically lagged with gypsum board.

Radiated sound is measured with the device suspended in the central area of the reverberant test room, and the connected inlet and discharge ductwork is heavy gauge sheet metal lagged with gypsum board or other enclosure materials and ducted outside the test room. However, if the unit has an air induction inlet, this is left exposed within the test room.

ARI Standard 880-94 specifies several pressure and air flows for rating the unit. The ARI certification program entails annual check tests on randomly selected samples of participating manufacturers' products and the publication of a directory of performance for "certified units." At present, the ratings are for both discharge and radiated sound at the single operating point of 1.5 in. w.g. inlet static pressure and nominal 2000 fpm inlet velocity for most product types but include fan-only conditions for fan-powered terminals.

Many manufacturers also catalog, or make available upon request, octave-band sound power level data at operating points other than the one used for ARI certification. These points are usually derived by testing at a sufficient number of different operating points to develop a reliable estimation procedure based upon a multiple variable regression analysis of the test data.

TESTING IN A MOCK-UP INSTALLATION

Some acoustical consultants, engineers, and developers require full-scale mock-up testing, sometimes referred to as an "in situ" test. In most cases, the test space is configured in a realistic manner, incorporating the proposed ceiling system, a typical plenum depth (36 in. deep, unbounded at the sides above the room walls), and a representative room size. So many tests have been conducted in rooms with a nominal 2400 ft^3 volume (200 ft^2 to 250 ft^2 of floor area depending upon the effective ceiling height) that this physical size is becoming a "de facto" standard.

Octave-band sound pressure level measurements are usually made in such a mock-up facility at a point directly beneath the air terminal, about 5 ft above the floor. This is usually a worst case situation. (The *ARI Standard 885-90 Applications Procedure* recommends the space average of four locations in the room, but this is seldom followed in most instances.) The measured sound pressure levels are then usually converted to a simplified NC rating and evaluated on a pass/fail basis. (See Chapter 3 for a description of how NC ratings are determined.) The RC sound descriptor is becoming more important in order to evaluate, to some degree, sound quality issues.

UNCERTAINTIES IN THE APPLICATION OF MANUFACTURERS' DATA

The possible uncertainties in the application of manufacturers' data for air terminal units are provided in Table 11-1. These are based upon utilized test standards and results found in testing programs.

TABLE 11-1
Estimated Variability of Sound Power Data and Bands Most Affected by System Effects

Air Terminal Units, Fan Powered Mixing, Shut-Off VAV Boxes						
Octave Mid-Band Frequency	Measurement Uncertainty of Std. Test Procedure[a] dB	Repeatability of Test Data[b] dB	Production Variability[c] dB	Cumulative Uncer-tainty Due To All Previous Factors[d] dB	Variability of Random Sample *re* Catalog[e] dB	Bands Most Affected by System Effects[f]
63	*[g]	*	*	*	*	*
125	± 3 dB	± 2 dB	+5, -2 dB	± 6 dB	+5, -2 dB	+5 dB
250	± 2 dB	± 2 dB	± 4 dB	± 5 dB	± 4 dB	+5 dB
500-4000	± 1.5 dB	± 1 dB	± 3 dB	± 3 dB	± 3 dB	
8000	± 3 dB	± 2 dB	± 3 dB	± 5 dB	± 3 dB	

a. Based on ANSI S12-31 for pure tones and assumes that the expected range is one standard deviation.
b. Repetitive testing of same unit in same laboratory.
c. Subject to manufacturing tolerances permitted in quality control.
d. Based on the square root of the sum of the squares of all uncertainties.
e. Fan-powered units have higher variability than shut-off VAV units due to differences from fan motors.
f. See discussion of system effects earlier in this chapter.
g. No test procedures are in place to determine 63 Hz data for these products.

APPLICATION OF AIR TERMINAL ACOUSTICAL DATA TO BUILDING SYSTEMS

The presentation of air terminal application data is not currently specified by any standard, although application guidelines are provided in ARI Standard 885-90. Most manufacturers present simplified estimated NC ratings based upon whatever room conversion factors they deem appropriate. Most manufacturers are also using the guidelines provided in ARI Standard 885-90, which is presently the most comprehensive source of available information on the appropriate conversion from sound power level to room sound pressure level for air terminal devices.

Since manufacturers are presently free to choose whatever application factors they desire, there is little commonality among suppliers. Although most manufacturers may state what assumptions were used in converting the product sound power level data to the simplified single-number NC rating, it must be recognized that these assumptions are not always appropriate to the application.

Manufacturers are subjected to strong marketing pressures to present data in as favorable a light as possible but not necessarily at the most realistic conditions. Such marketing-driven uses of the available knowledge have become so prevalent that ARI is considering proposals to standardize application assumptions.

RECOMMENDED DESIGN AND INSTALLATION PRACTICES FOR AIR TERMINAL DEVICES

Following are problems common to all types of VAV air terminal devices.

INLET CONDITIONS

- Poor inlet conditions (such as sharp bends or manual damper immediately before the unit, as illustrated in Figure 11-1) can cause significant errors in the sensed airflow through the unit. If these conditions exist within one equivalent diameter, the sensed flow can be significantly in error (20% or more) and result in more than the desired flow through the unit. This results in higher sound levels than predicted for both the box and the diffusers downstream.
- If flexible duct is used at the inlet, it is virtually acoustically transparent and can result in higher than predicted radiated sound beneath the unit. This occurs because the sound power generated by the damper in the terminal device is transmitted in both directions from the unit and can break out through the transparent walls of flexible inlet ductwork. While this is seldom a problem, when inlet pressures exceed 2 in. w.g. and inlet ducts are 12 in. diameter, larger breakout noise may become significant. Breakout noise at the inlet to a unit is not presently covered in any application guides or standards.
- A sharp bend in the duct at the inlet can also generate significant noise.

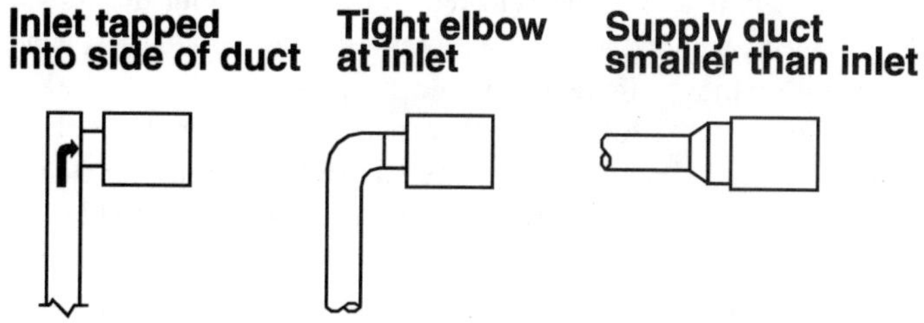

FIGURE 11-1 Inlet effects.

Solution

Provide as little flexible duct at the inlet as possible; make it straight and keep air velocities well below 2000 fpm to minimize regenerated noise. However, if ductwork upstream of the branch takeoff is not acoustically lined, the insulated flexible duct may offer the only acoustical attenuation of upstream noise. Thus, this is somewhat of a catch-22 situation when inlet static pressures exceed 2 in. w.g.

Outlet Conditions

A poor aerodynamic configuration at the unit outlet can generate excessive noise. Tee fittings too close to a terminal can create additional radiated and ductborne noise due to excessive turbulence. The discharge air-velocity profile from fan-powered units interacting with a close-coupled downstream balancing damper can create localized areas of high turbulence and increased noise generation.

Solution

Several duct diameters of straight duct (preferably lined) should be provided before any abrupt transitions, bends, or splits to allow the discharge flow profile to expand and fill the duct, minimizing potential regenerated noise.

Vibration Isolation

Air terminals seldom require external vibration isolation. Most fan-powered units have some form of internal motor isolation included as part of the packaged design.

Product Sizing

In general, at a given flow rate, a larger unit will be quieter than a smaller unit. There are several problems with over-sizing units, however. Units should be selected to operate within the manufacturer's recommended airflow and pressure ranges, with best acoustical results achieved in the maximum range of 1500 fpm to 1800 fpm inlet velocity at the full-design flow rate. Primary-air inlet velocities below 300 fpm generally cannot be controlled well as the flow sensors and transducers used become unreliable. Fans throttled to operate at airflow below their normal capacity range may surge or stall. If the speed is lowered below about 600 rpm, reduced bearing life will occur because of a lack of reliable lubrication when sleeve bearings are used. Also, electric heaters can present problems with minimum velocities where overheating of the heating elements may occur when oversized units are used.

On the other hand, inlet duct velocities above about 2500 fpm can result in high self-generated inlet noise, high pressure loss, and may exceed the flow sensor's maximum range of control.

Solution

Select units that are in the middle of their published operation range with around two-thirds of rated airflow rate and 2 in. wc inlet static pressure being recommended upper operating limits.

Variations in Room Sound Level

In VAV applications, room sound levels due to air terminal devices will vary as a function of the airflow necessary to handle the thermal load. When the thermal load is nominally constant, as in most interior spaces, the room sound level is also relatively constant. However, when the thermal load varies, the room sound level varies as well. This is most noticeable in perimeter spaces as the sun moves across a building during the daytime. Areas exposed to the sun have not only the highest thermal loads, but also the highest sound levels. When units are selected to meet the design noise criteria under peak load conditions, the reduced air delivery at lower thermal loads may result in the loss of beneficial masking background noise with a corresponding degradation in the quality of speech privacy perceived in the environment.

Solution

Series-flow (constant-volume) fan-powered terminals often can be used to minimize the impact of a loss in speech privacy at reduced thermal loading. This is possible because both the air volume circulating in the external system and the sound generation of the unit are relatively constant. However, when the quality of speech privacy is a critical factor in the room-acoustics design, the use of a separate electronic sound-masking system provides the best assurance of meeting the specified requirements. Note that while these terminals are constant volume discharge, the inlet primary air usually uses a VAV valve or damper with the balance of the air provided by the induction air port.

OTHER PRACTICAL NOISE CONTROL OPTIONS

- Maintain the lowest practical duct static pressure.
- Maintain duct static pressures as constant as possible. Dampers and orifice plates installed upstream of VAV air terminals to reduce high duct pressures at branch takeoffs near the supply fan can reduce the operating static pressure of the unit and, thus, reduce the sound level at rated airflow. Such pressure reduction devices should not be located closer than five duct diameters upstream of the unit to avoid introducing errors in the terminal's inlet velocity sensor. However, it must be pointed out that the pressure reduction across dampers and orifice plates at branch takeoff varies with the square of the velocity of through-flow. Therefore, at low airflow through the VAV terminal, nearly the full pressure in the main duct may be present at the box inlet because the external pressure reduction devices cease to be effective.
- If discharge noise is a problem, or if there is no lining downstream of the terminal, the addition of about 5 ft of nonmetallic core insulated flexible duct at each diffuser outlet can often serve as a flexible sound attenuator. Flexible duct is generally overlooked as a potential noise reduction device because acoustical performance data are not commonly available. However, insertion loss and breakout factors for typical nonmetallic core fiberglass insulated flexible duct are currently listed in ARI Standard 885-90. In the application of flexible duct, it is important to ensure that the installation is as straight as possible; badly kinked flexible duct can add significant pressure drop and self-generated noise to the system.
- If radiated noise is a problem in units without induction ports, lagging the box, and the first few feet downstream with drywall, using a construction adhesive and screws on 6 in. centers is sometimes effective (refer to Figure 5-5 for a more detailed description). The relative effectiveness of this lagging is greatest on the larger-size units because the area around the controls that cannot be lagged is a smaller percentage of the total exposed surface area. However, such lagging treatment is not beneficial on units having induction ports because the amount of sound radiated directly through these ports is usually significantly greater than that radiated by the box casing. Try to locate the unit away from open return air grilles.

- Whenever possible, utilize lined ductwork, flexible duct, and multiple branches downstream of the terminal device. Try to maintain at least 2 to 3 diameters of lined duct downstream of the boxes before making the first diffuser takeoff. Use rigid round ductwork upstream of the terminal device.
- Avoid the location of fan-powered or air-to-air induction terminals in regions directly above acoustically sensitive spaces when low background noise is desired.

Fan Speed Control

Fan-powered air terminals with a fan-speed controller will modulate air volume much more quietly than those with damper controls. Almost all series and parallel fan-powered air terminals have a fan speed controller installed as a standard feature. However, it is most important to ensure that the speed controller and motor are properly matched by the manufacturer because at low rpms, excessive motor hum (typically pure tones at 120 Hz and higher harmonics) may result if the combination is mismatched. In addition, at motor speeds of 600 rpm or less, the centrifugally lubricated sleeve bearings used on most units will have a shortened life due to insufficient lubrication.

Flow Sensors

Duct pressures change in VAV systems in response to changing load requirements throughout the building. In order for VAV air terminals to operate independently of any inlet pressure variations (called pressure-independent operation), they require flow sensors in the unit to measure actual flow rates and signal the controller to regulate the damper position. A side benefit of pressure independence is a much more stable acoustical performance.

The flow sensor, however, is not without problems. It generates both additional pressure drop and noise. A sensor with optimum accuracy at low flow rates (where the unit is the most quiet) often has higher self-generated sound and pressure losses at the higher airflow volumes. Any flow sensor design must make a compromise between pressure drop, noise, and signal strength. Flow-averaging probes are used to allow operation at less than ideal inlet conditions and at lower airflow than a pitot tube-type sensor. Thus, changing the type of inlet sensor can significantly affect the sound generation of a unit. ARI certified units are required to have the most common type of flow sensor device installed when rating the unit. Special controls, however, may require special inlet sensors, and this is a factor to consider in an acoustically critical application. When in doubt, always specify that the submitted sound data be obtained with the flow probe to be used on the project installed.

Effect of Controls on Noise

The types of controls used on an air terminal device may affect the resulting sound level in the receiving space.

- Different control types have differing minimum flow capabilities. Pneumatic-type, true proportional, continuous signal/response controls are often better at controlling low flow rates than most digital controllers, whose typical response at the low end tends to be a step function (often with surprisingly large steps). As airflow varies at minimum conditions, sound levels will also vary. More importantly, air pressures in the ductwork near the unit can be caused to fluctuate, creating noise fluctuations in adjacent units.
- The minimum capabilities of different types of controls can affect the selection of unit sizes. For example, a pneumatic unit can be selected one size larger than a DDC (direct digital control) unit when controlling at the desired minimum value. This will result in quieter comparative performance at the higher airflow.
- Some analog electronic and DDC controls have the capability of varying the fan speed in fan-powered air terminals. Thus, by maintaining the fan speed as low as possible, reduced noise generation will be present.

In summary, both the acoustical signature and the selection process of VAV air terminals are affected by the control selection of a unit.

External Ductwork Considerations

Inadequate Length Downstream of Fan-Powered Terminals

Very short diffuser distribution plenums downstream of fan-powered air terminals can result in fan instability in the form of stall or surge. The fan is located on the discharge side of many fan-powered units, and several diameters of downstream duct are required to achieve low-turbulent, properly established, and stable airflow. If an abrupt transition occurs before fully developed airflow is established, the excessive turbulence created results in a fluctuating discharge pressure seen by the fan, which is sufficient in some cases to cause the fan to become unstable. Significant problems of this nature occur in many retrofit applications where adequate space to obtain fully developed airflow downstream of the fan is unavailable. As a consequence, fan surge is frequently encountered, and this affects not only the air performance, but introduces annoying, fluctuating sound levels in the receiving room.

Indoor Air Quality (IAQ) Impact on Noise

The use of glass-fiber and other porous duct-lining materials has become an important concern with regard to indoor air quality (IAQ). Porous materials, if allowed to become dirty within a high relative humidity environment, become an ideal breeding ground for microbial growth. Although ASHRAE is presently developing HVAC system design guidelines to minimize this potential problem, the current trend, driven by IAQ concerns, is often to eliminate the use of porous, acoustically absorbent duct-lining materials in air distribution systems. This has a significant impact on the system noise level coupled to the receiving space through air terminal devices and outlets. As a result, the elimination of porous, acoustically absorbent duct liner materials significantly impacts the system designer and component manufacturers who must jointly find new methods for coping with up to 20 dB higher system noise levels than encountered at the present time. Hopefully, there is a rational solution to this potential problem that will not require the complete elimination of acoustically absorbent materials in all areas of the air distribution system. One possibility is to use facing materials of plastic or metal-foil sheeting to protect the porous surface from direct exposure to the airstream. The disadvantage is that such facings, unless they are very thin, will substantially degrade the acoustical efficiency in the mid- to high-frequency region, where the need for sound absorption is the greatest!

These concerns have been seen to produce serious sources of noise problems in regions of the country with high humidity climates. Often, the noise problems have not been discovered until after commissioning and building occupancy where remedial noise control solutions are difficult to find and often expensive to put into place. In-line duct silencers are often tried with less than desired results with the introduction of self-noise generation by the silencers.

Ceiling Plenum Effects

The combined acoustical effects of a suspended ceiling, with a typical plenum space above, has been empirically developed from in situ tests, conducted primarily on fan-powered terminals, in several industry mock-up facilities. The results are incorporated in tabular form in ARI Standard 885-90. A number of acoustically sensitive projects using fan-powered terminals have been successfully installed based on the procedures recommended in this application standard.

However, recent research funded by ASHRAE (Warnock 1998a, 1998b, 1998c) suggests that some terminal types, other than fan-powered boxes, may require different attenuation factors to convert from the product sound power level, determined in a reverberant test facility, to room sound pressure level in a typical receiving room environment. These recently completed research study results have not been sufficiently analyzed to the extent that new application guidelines have yet been formulated. Until this is resolved, a full-scale mock-up is still the best alternative in critical situations.

SPECIFIC AIR TERMINAL APPLICATION NOISE CHARACTERISTICS

Reheat Air Terminals

VAV air terminals often have factory-supplied attached hot water or electric coils to raise the temperature of the air supplied to the space, as illustrated in Figure 11-2. The acoustical implications of these devices include the following.

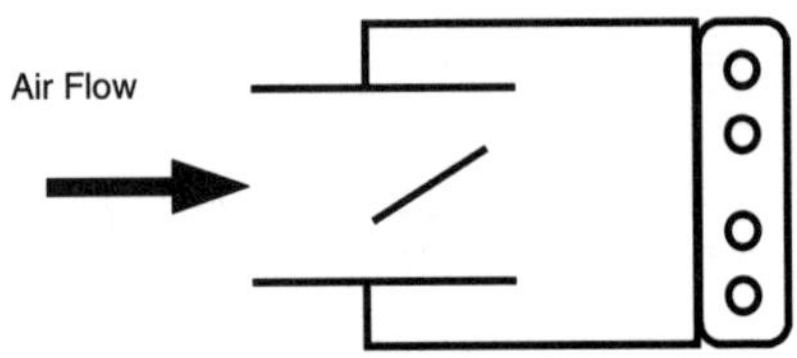

FIGURE 11-2 VAV terminal with reheat coil.

Water Coils

Because of the additional pressure drop introduced by the presence of water coils, the pressure drop across the control damper of a VAV unit that is required to obtain the desired flow volume is reduced. This typically reduces the damper-generated noise for a given pressure in the inlet duct. Water coils, themselves, seldom produce regenerated noise unless they are mismatched in size to the attached VAV unit. The beneficial effect of water coils attached to a VAV unit is not routinely reported in manufacturers' acoustical data.

Electric Heat Units

Electric heating coils typically have little acoustical effect. However, electric heater air distribution baffles, which can introduce a pressure drop, are installed to equalize airflow across the heating coils. Although the baffles may generate some additional noise, this tends to be offset by the lower pressure drop required across the unit. Thus, damper-generated noise is reduced. In many cases, electric heat equipped units must be greater in length to comply with code restrictions imposed upon damper location upstream of heating elements. Consequently, these units are usually quieter than standard units because of a greater length of integral acoustically lined duct.

DUAL-DUCT AIR TERMINALS

These units are used to mix two different streams of air flowing into a common outlet duct, as illustrated in Figure 11-3. Because there is considerably more exposed sheet metal area in dual-duct units, the radiated sound is usually higher than that of an equivalent single-duct unit.

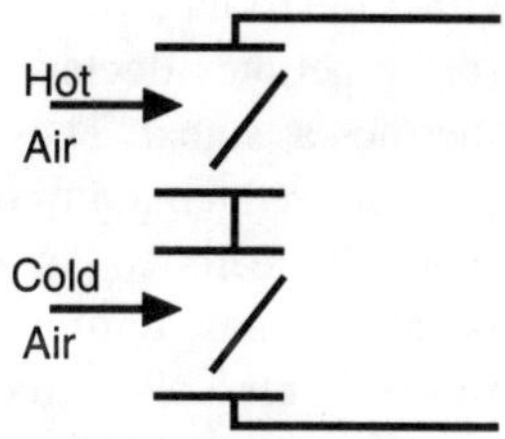

FIGURE 11-3 Dual-duct air terminals.

Acoustical data are seldom provided for the combined flow because it is not covered in the present test procedures. However, it can be calculated by logarithmic summation of the contributions of each inlet duct. The worst case condition is typically when one inlet is furnishing the full design airflow at the maximum expected inlet static pressure.

A discharge mixer, as illustrated in Figure 11-4, if supplied, will add increased pressure drop and alter unit sound levels. The increased pressure drop will lower valve-generated sound by reducing the

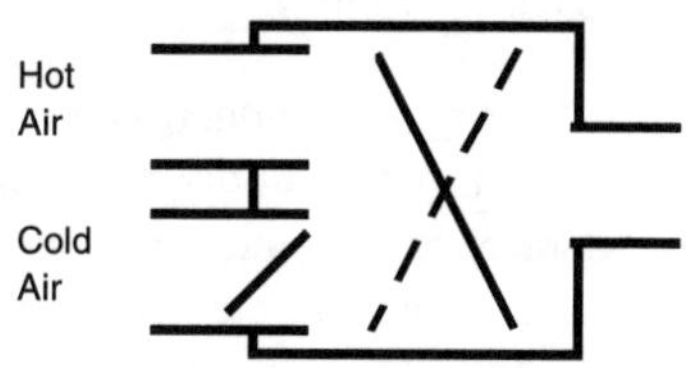

FIGURE 11-4 Dual duct with mixers.

velocity across the damper for a given inlet pressure. The mixer will tend to introduce some self-generated noise, but if factory fabricated, acoustical data should be available. However, if field installed, this factor will be an unknown.

BYPASS UNITS

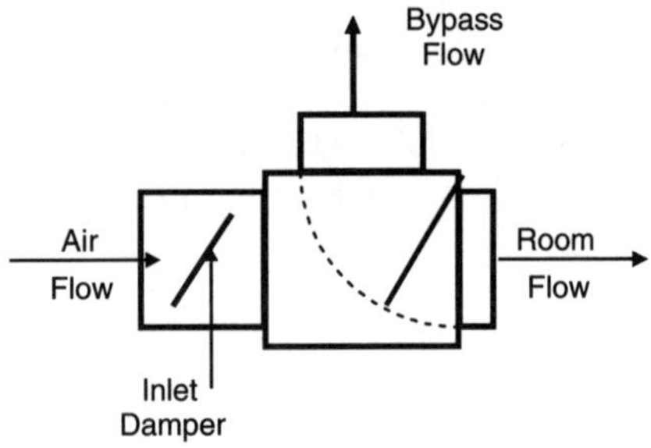

FIGURE 11-5 Bypass units.

Bypass units, as illustrated in Figure 11-5, are not truly VAV boxes in the sense of the commonly accepted definition because they do not vary the quantity of air delivered by the system supply fan. They are used in conjunction with constant-volume systems where variable volume air delivery to a particular zone is desired. Supply air is directed to either the room diffusers or partially bypassed to the ceiling plenum (or sometimes ducted back to the central fan) in proportion to a thermostat signal. These units are not intended to be used as VAV/ pressure-reducing air control devices, although they often are. This typically leads to an early damper failure and noise problems because bypass terminals are often rated at much lower inlet velocities and pressures than conventional VAV air terminals.

If a bypass unit is not properly installed or balanced, both acoustical and flow control problems will result. Bypass units used at airflow exceeding the manufacturer's nominally rated flow (typically 1500 fpm maximum) or inlet pressure (typically 0.3 in. wc) may actually fail in operation. In general, even at rated airflow rates and pressures, bypass units generate significantly more sound than typical VAV terminals.

AIR-TO-AIR INDUCTION AIR TERMINALS

Air-to-air induction air terminals are employed to mix plenum air with cold supply air using the velocity pressure in the supply duct nozzle to induce plenum air, providing a nearly constant airflow with variable temperature to the space without mechanical mixing. This design requires fairly high inlet duct pressures to develop the velocity necessary for adequate induction. At least one port is open to the plenum to obtain the induction air. As a result, the potential for radiated noise problems is fairly great, and care must be taken in the selection and location of these units to minimize complaints.

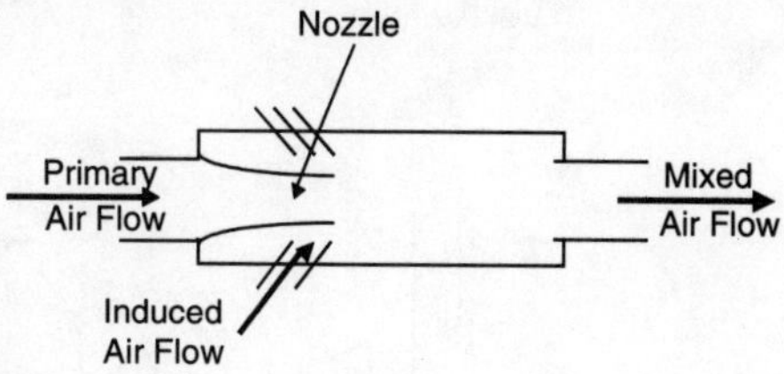

FIGURE 11-6 Air-to-air induction terminal.

FAN-POWERED AIR TERMINALS

These units are available in both parallel (variable airflow, "side pocket") and (constant airflow) series flow versions. These air terminals can create low-frequency noise problems when located above sensitive occupied spaces.

Parallel, VAV Fan-Powered Air Terminals

Parallel air terminals, as illustrated in Figure 11-7, deliver a varying flow volume to the room in the cooling mode and a constant flow volume in the heating mode. The fan is typically sized to supply about one-half the VAV maximum primary airflow volume, and the level of fan noise is often less than with a comparable series flow terminal. The most significant problem with noise occurs when the fan starts on demand for heat to the space and the character of sound noticeably changes. Sound attenuators installed on the induction inlet port are sometimes effective with parallel units because the sound escaping from the inlet port usually dominates that of the direct casing radiated noise.

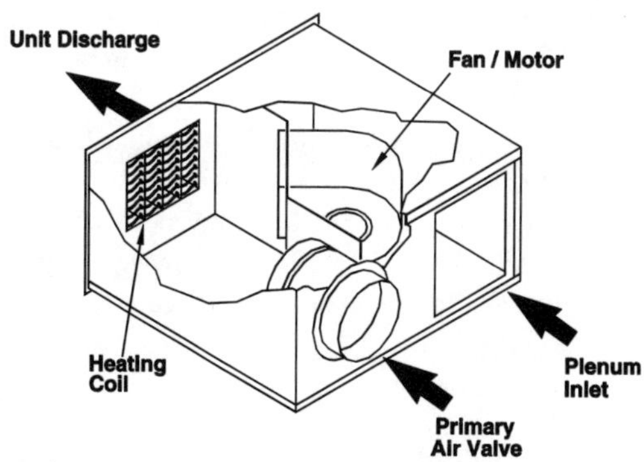

FIGURE 11-7 Parallel, VAV fan-powered air terminal.

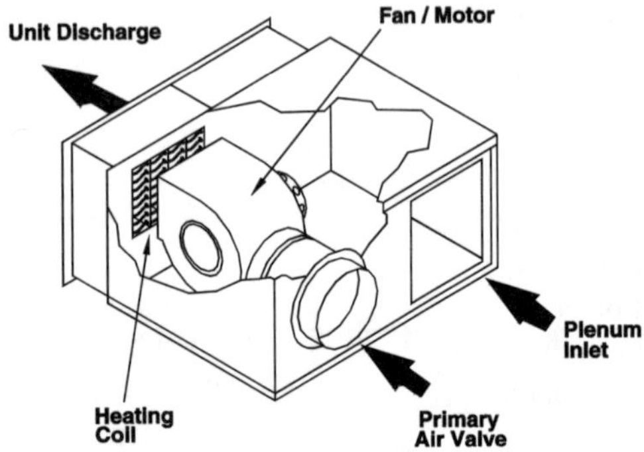

FIGURE 11-8 Series flow, constant-volume, fan-powered air terminal.

Series Flow, Constant-Volume, Fan-Powered Air Terminals

In series flow air terminals, the fan operates continuously whenever air is delivered to the room. As illustrated in Figure 11-8, the fan is located at or near the discharge of the unit. Consequently, the level of discharge noise is relatively constant, as is the airflow rate, regardless of the thermal load. When acoustically lined duct is used following the unit discharge, excessive noise is seldom a problem. However, applications that do not permit the use of downstream duct liner frequently experience problems with excessive discharge noise.

Radiated sound levels vary significantly with variations in both duct pressure and thermal load. Attempts to quiet the sound radiating from the induction port with attenuators are seldom successful because the added pressure drop requires an increase in fan speed to restore air delivery, and this essentially offsets any anticipated benefit. Another effect of adding inlet sound attenuators (and with some quiet designs) is a condition sometimes referred to as *fan shift*. This is a condition where the unit delivers more air when in the full-cooling mode than when in either the partial cooling or heating mode. If the induction port offers a significant restriction to induced airflow, then there will be a change in airflow to the room when the primary valve varies from minimum to maximum flow rate. This can cause objectionable changes in diffuser noise levels as thermal loads change.

Series fan air terminals are usually equipped with a low-cost silicon-controlled rectifier (SCR) speed controller installed in the unit for balancing purposes. The SCR device is usually a "chopper" type of speed controller that reduces the fan speed and, thus, fan-generated noise but has the potential of increasing motor hum if the motor and speed controller are not matched properly. This can produce annoying tonal components at 120 Hz and higher harmonics that are difficult to attenuate.

If fan speed is lowered much below 600 rpm, excessive motor bearing wear will result. Also, if the start-up sequence allows primary air to enter the unit prior to fan start, the unit may have insufficient start-up torque to overcome the tendency for these units to rotate backwards. It is not uncommon to discover that series boxes have been oversized for the application as a result of a desire for quiet operation. The reduced airflow further causes the motors to run hotter, reducing expected motor life, and thereby increasing operational costs.

Low-Profile Fan-Powered Air Terminals

Low-profile fan-powered air terminals are available in both parallel and series types. Usually designed to have an installed height no greater than 10.5 in., these air terminals have limited capacity if compared to the more typical taller versions. When installed in shallow rather than in the typical 3 ft depth plenum spaces, the radiated noise via the ceiling path can be significantly increased.

Retrofit Air Terminals

Many manufacturers offer a number of solutions for retrofitting existing systems. There are four general types; each has unique acoustical characteristics and are difficult to predict. In most cases, these devices are used to operate at lower system pressures than originally required (to reduce energy costs) and result in reduced noise levels.

- *Type 1: Internally-mounted, design specific, mechanical constant-volume replacement units.* These are custom designed to replace specific high-pressure mechanical dampers with externally-powered (electric or pneumatic) VAV dampers.
- *Type 2: Externally-mounted VAV conversion units.* These are add-on units, typically round ducts with internal dampers and flow sensors, that are added at the inlet of existing units and are then gutted of their mechanical flow controllers. The old unit casings then act as mixers or sound attenuators.
- *Type 3: Slip-in add-on VAV damper.* Designed to be slid into

existing ductwork, these are designed to add a VAV control zone where one did not exist before.

- *Type 4: Sleeve-type VAV dampers.* These are essentially a section of duct with an installed VAV damper and flow sensor. Used in both new and existing buildings, these are custom made to fit the application.

SUGGESTED SPECIFICATIONS FOR AIR TERMINALS

An ideal specification for air terminals should specify the octave-band sound power level limit spectrum at design static pressure and include a statement of the factors to be used in conversion from sound power level to room sound pressure level. The specification should also specify the room noise criterion used as the basis for system design. The use of *ARI Standard 885-90, Procedure for Estimating Occupied Space Sound Levels in the Application of Air Terminals and Air Outlets* is recommended for guidance in establishing realistic sound power to sound pressure conversion factors.

It is important to understand that the design room noise criterion applies to the system as a whole and only indirectly to the noise produced by the specified component. However, it follows that the contribution of the component to the total system noise in the room cannot exceed the spectrum of the specified room noise criterion at any point. Thus, there are two ways to develop a specification for air terminal devices.

- The first is to specify the maximum octave-band sound power levels of the unit by working backwards from the design room sound pressure level criterion for the system as a whole and adding the conversion factors from sound pressure to sound power level using the guidelines recommended in ARI Standard 885-90.
- The second method is to specify the system design room sound pressure level criterion and make a unit selection based on the manufacturer's catalog ratings that have been derived by using suggested default factors provided in ARI Standard 885-90.

The second method is easier for the specifying engineer to use, but its reliability depends upon how close the default conversion values used match the details of the intended application. Therefore, it is essential that the manufacturer clearly list the assumptions made in cataloging unit performance in terms of room sound pressure level noise criteria.

For example, the following factors must be considered in cataloging the acoustical performance of a VAV air terminal device for discharge noise:

1. The total number of air outlets served by the terminal device
2. The number of these outlets serving a typical room
3. The dimensions of this typical room
4. The length and dimensions of acoustically lined duct downstream of the unit discharge
5. The size and typical length of flexible branch duct connected to an air outlet
6. The specified room noise criterion to be met
7. The location in the room where the specified room noise criterion is to be qualified

The following factors must be considered in cataloging the performance of a VAV air terminal device for casing and induction port (when present) radiated noise:

1. The height of the ceiling plenum
2. The type of ceiling beneath the unit
3. The dimensions of the room beneath the unit
4. The size of any openings in the ceiling for plenum return, if any
5. The specified room noise criterion to be met
6. The location in the room where the specified room noise criterion is to be qualified

The logarithmic addition of the discharge and radiated sound in the room, attributable to the air terminal device, will establish whether or not the unit meets the specified design room noise criterion. The criterion is met if this addition results in octave-band sound pressure levels that do not exceed the spectrum of the specified criterion at any point.

An example of the first method, backward calculation, follows.

VAV Terminal Sound/Pressure Specification

Project Guide Specification for Manufacturers' Sound Data

The pressure drop through the units shall not exceed scheduled values, including hot water coils. The unit manufacturer shall furnish certified sound data for both casing radiated and discharge sound levels as tested per ARI Industry Standard 880-94. Both discharge and radiated sound shall result in room sound pressure levels not to exceed those listed below, with a tolerance of +2 dB in any band for less than 20% of the units. The sound pressure shall be determined in accordance with ARI 885-90 from certified sound power levels determined in accordance with ARI 880-94, with the listed assumptions:

Select desired noise criteria

- Desired room sound pressure level (dB) by octave bands to meet project:
  For a design sound criteria with RC of 40(N),

	Octave Band Mid-Band Frequency (Hz)					
	125	250	500	1000	2000	4000
Desired Room Sound Pressure Level (dB):	60	55	45	40	35	33

Application assumptions

- Nominal terminal unit inlet size is 12 in. diameter,
- Nominal duct inlet static pressure is 1.0 in. wc, and
- Environmental adjustment factor is to be used (see ARI 885-90 for discussion).

Discharge sound

- Sound power division based on 5 ft of acoustically lined duct,
- Two power splits or divisions,
- Five feet of 8 in. diameter flexible duct to each diffusers, and
- End reflection based on an 8 in. diameter round duct.

Radiated sound

- ADC/ARI Standard 885, ceiling/plenum with no duct breakout:

	Octave Band Mid-Band Frequency (Hz)					
	125	250	500	1000	2000	4000
Ceiling/Plenum Attenuation (dB):	9	10	12	14	15	15

- Room absorption based on a 2400 ft^3 room, 5 ft from the source:

	Octave Band Mid-Band Frequency (Hz)					
	125	250	500	1000	2000	4000
Room Effect (dB):	5	7	8	9	10	11

Maximum sound power level

Based on these assumptions, neither the unit radiated nor discharge sound power levels shall exceed the following levels at an inlet static pressure of 1.0 in. wc.

Both radiated and discharge sound power levels shall be based on the most current ARI Certified data, as reflected in the most current Certified Product Directory.

Octave Bands (Hz)	125	250	500	1000	2000	4000
Radiated L_w (dB)	77	74	66	64	61	60
Discharge L_w (dB)	83	81	79	87	85	68

REFERENCES

Warnock, A.C.C. 1998a. Environmental correction factors for predicting room sound pressure levels. *ASHRAE Transactions* 104(1A): 638.

Warnock, A.C.C. 1998b. Sound pressure level vs. distance from sources in rooms. *ASHRAE Transactions* 104(1A): 643.

Warnock, A.C.C. 1998c. Transmission of sound from air terminal devices through ceiling systems. *ASHRAE Transactions* 104(1A): 650.

Chapter 12
Room Fan Coil Units

by *Warren Blazier*

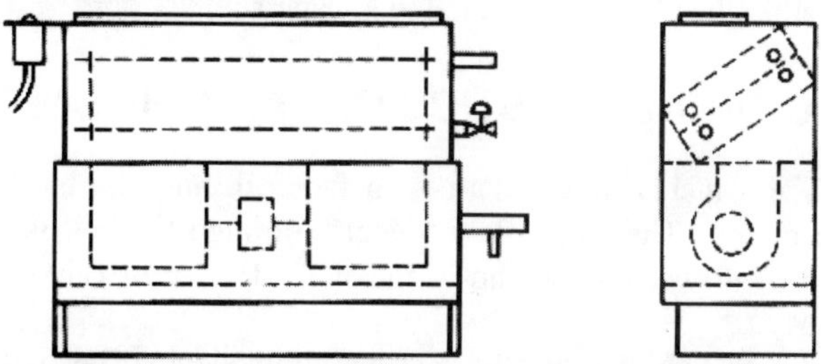

OVERVIEW

Room fan coil units are typically nonducted, packaged cooling and heating equipment designed to provide air conditioning in individual spaces such as hotel and motel rooms, private or semi-private offices, etc., not served by a central air distribution system. They are also used in perimeter areas of open-plan spaces in buildings to handle the thermal loads associated with exterior environmental conditions. A fan coil unit is composed of a finned-tube coil through which conditioned water is circulated, a fan section with a direct-drive motor, and an air filter. The fans are typically of the forward-curved type and driven by manually selected three-speed motors or motors with adjustable speed SCR controllers. During the cooling function, the fan continuously recirculates air from the space through the coil that is served by a remote source of chilled water. During the heating function, the coil is either served by a remote source of hot water or deactivated and replaced by an electrical resistance heating element. Room fan coil units typically range in size from 300 cfm to 1200 cfm. In general, fan coil units are available in three configurations:

1. Free-standing, low-profile horizontal units designed for use under windows with low sills
2. Vertical floor-to-ceiling units, chase-enclosed
3. Horizontal overhead units designed for installation in furred-down ceilings in spaces such as entrance vestibules or bathrooms in hotel/motel suites and meeting rooms. In these applications, a short discharge duct is generally connected to the unit

A second type of room fan coil unit is the indoor component of a duct-free split system, which is the matched combination of an outdoor condensing unit and a decorative indoor fan coil unit. In this case, the indoor coil is part of a direct-expansion refrigerant circuit rather than being connected to a water source.

NOISE CHARACTERISTICS OF FAN COIL UNITS

The principal noise sources in fan coil units are the fan and drive motor. (The water flow velocity through the coil is usually low enough that noise is not a factor if the control valve is sized properly.)

The fan noise typically has two components. The first is the non-tonal, distributed broad-band noise, subjectively perceived as a rumble, roar, or hiss, depending upon where the fan is operating on its air performance curve. The second is a tonal component produced at the blade-passage frequency of the fan wheel (number of fan blades × rpm/60). This typically is perceived as a whine and occurs in the frequency range of 500 Hz to 1000 Hz, depending upon the fan speed. The amplitude of this tone depends upon the clearance between the wheel and the cutoff of the fan scroll. "Tight" scroll configurations are the noisiest.

The motor noise is principally tonal in character. The most predominant tones occur at the twice-line frequency of 120 Hz and harmonics (100 Hz with 50 cps power) and are subjectively perceived as a hum or buzz, depending upon the harmonic structure. The hum or buzz may also be both amplitude and frequency-modulated at the slip-rate of the motor. The noise level of these tonal components depends upon motor type, quality, and the effectiveness of vibration isolation provided between the motor mounting and the equipment frame. With SCR drives, the "cleanness" of the electrical waveform supplied the motor by the speed controller to a large extent governs the generation of other annoying tonal components of motor noise.

Tap-wound motors tend to be significantly quieter than those whose speed is controlled by a solid-state device.

SOUND STANDARDS AND DATA AVAILABILITY

ARI is the cognizant industry association for the development of sound rating standards for room fan coil equipment, including the indoor component of a duct-free split system. The current standard for sound rating these units is *ARI 350-86, Sound Rating of Non-Ducted Indoor Air-Conditioning Equipment.*

UNCERTAINTIES IN SOUND RATING DATA

The standard for obtaining sound data on room fan coil units requires a reverberant-room test facility. The accuracy achievable is a function of the test room size and its acoustical design. There are other factors as well that can affect the reliability of data. Table 12-1 lists the uncertainties in the field application of manufacturers' data.

TABLE 12-1
Estimated Variability of Product Sound Power Data Due to Measurement Uncertainties and Production Quality Control

Room Fan Coil Units					
Octave Mid-Band Frequency Hz	Measurement Uncertainty of Std. Test Procedure[a] dB	Repeatability of Test Data[b] dB	Production Variability[c] dB	Cumulative Uncertainty Due To All Previous Factors[d] dB	Variability of Random Sample *re* Catalog[e] dB
63	± 4 dB	± 2 dB	± 4 dB	± 6 dB	+6, -0 dB
125	± 3 dB	± 1 dB	± 3 dB	± 4 dB	+5, -0 dB
250	± 2 dB	± 1 dB	± 3 dB	± 4 dB	+3, -0 dB
500-4000	± 1.5 dB	± 1 dB	± 3 dB	± 4 dB	+3, -0 dB
8000	± 3 dB	± 0.5 dB	± 3 dB	± 4 dB	+3, -0 dB

a. Standard deviation of octave-band data per ISO 3741.
b. Repetitive testing of same unit in same laboratory.
c. Subject to manufacturing tolerances permitted in production quality control.
d. Based on the square root of the sum of the squares of all uncertainties.
e. Published catalog data are not customarily derived from a statistical sampling of production units but usually are determined by testing a prototype. Thus, the results of testing random production samples would tend to exceed those published by the manufacturer.

ARI Standard Sound Rating Number (SR_{ARI})

The ARI sound rating (SR_{ARI}) is stated as a single number, the A-weighted sound power level expressed in bels. (Bels are used to avoid confusion with the A-weighted sound pressure level, which is expressed in decibels. One bel equals ten decibels.) The first step in the test procedure requires determining the sound power level spectrum of the product noise source in one-third octave bands. This provides 21 pieces of data about the spectral characteristics of the noise source. The second step is to subject these data to a complicated correction procedure to adjust for irregularities in the spectrum, presumably to account for tonal content. The final step is to process the "corrected" one-third octave-band spectrum to obtain the "tone-corrected" A-weighted sound power level, SR_{ARI}, which is the ARI sound rating number.

In application, this single number rating, SR_{ARI}, has little engineering significance, except as a basis for comparing unit A to B to C, etc. It cannot be used to predict the sound level produced in a room in which the product might be installed because it is not possible to make the conversion from source sound power level to room sound pressure level without knowledge of the frequency spectrum of the noise. The SR_{ARI} rating does not provide this information.

Furthermore, because the frequency structure of the noise is unknown, there is also no way to evaluate the subjective character of the noise (how it sounds to the ear). Although competitive units produced by different manufacturers might have equal ARI sound ratings, this does not mean that they would be judged equally noisy (or quiet) in the opinion of a listener. In reality, one unit might be perceived as objectionable because of a frequency imbalance or an annoying audible tonal content, whereas another might be perceived as a bland, well-balanced acceptable sound. The A-weighted metric is insensitive to such differences in sound quality.

Suggested Alternative to the ARI Sound Rating Number, (SR_{ARI})

As pointed out above, the SR_{ARI} has little engineering significance in product application because it is not possible to use it to estimate the sound pressure levels that will be produced in the environment of the application nor does it provide any clue to the presence of annoying tonal components in the spectrum. The alternative is to utilize the one-third octave-band sound power level data required by the ARI Standard 350-86 test procedure for use in calculating the sound rating number, SR_{ARI}. The one-third octave data will reveal the presence of undesirable tonal components. Furthermore, if the acoustical characteristics of the receiving environment are known, the one-third octave sound power levels can also be converted to octave-band sound pressure levels for comparison to noise criteria that are usually expressed on this basis.

VIBRATION ISOLATION CONSIDERATIONS

Because of the nature of the installation, free standing and vertical floor-mounted fan coil units do not lend themselves to external vibration isolation. Thus, acceptable room noise levels ordinarily cannot be achieved without some form of internal vibration isolation of the fan and drive-motor assembly being incorporated by the manufacturer in the product design. However, ceiling-suspended horizontal units should be isolated using external rubber-in-shear hangers.

RECOMMENDED DESIGN AND INSTALLATION PRACTICES

Room fan coil units are frequently a source of noise complaints. One reason is that the units are normally in close proximity to the occupant and easily identifiable as a source of disturbance if too loud or the character of the noise is annoying. The fact that both the fan and drive motor are so closely coupled to the receiving room (nonducted) makes it very difficult to find adequate space to introduce noise control measures to correct a complaint. Thus, the possibility that something can be done after the fact should a noise complaint occur is a risky proposition. This is particularly true of the free-standing, low-profile, horizontal fan coil units because there is virtually no available space. Although somewhat more space may be available for noise control treatments in the chase-enclosed vertical floor-to-ceiling or furred-in overhead horizontal units, it may be impractical to utilize without significantly affecting fan performance.

The operating speed of the fan has the greatest effect on the noise level produced by a fan coil unit. For example, at rated capacity, a typical free-standing, low-profile horizontal fan coil unit operates at a speed of about 1100 rpm (high-speed setting). Under these conditions, the resulting noise level in typical applications, such as hotel/motel rooms, private and semi-private offices, etc., generally will be on the order of 10 dB greater than the criterion normally assigned to such spaces. However, switching the fan to a lower speed, such as 750 rpm for example, reduces the capacity by about one-third but reduces the noise level about 9 dB.

Fan coil units are usually sized for worst-case design-day cooling at high fan speed. Therefore, a majority of the time the unit can likely achieve proper room cooling and an acceptable noise level when operated at a reduced speed. However, given a situation in which the unit is required to meet the specified noise criterion at full design capacity, the only solution is to oversize the unit. Although it is recognized that this represents a higher first-cost, and perhaps some architectural juggling to accommodate a slightly larger unit, there is really no other practical alternative.

SUGGESTED NOISE SPECIFICATIONS

Noise Specifications

It is recommended that the engineer avoid using the ARI sound rating, SR_{ARI}, as a basis for specifying the acoustical performance of room fan coil units. It could lead to an unacceptable application because of the "caveat emptor" nature of this overly simplified sound rating.

Fortunately, ARI Standard 350-86 requires the determination of sound power levels in one-third octave bands as a first step in the process of developing the SR_{ARI}. A procedure is also provided in the standard for converting the one-third octave data to octave-band levels. Thus, two sets of product sound data of different resolution should be available from manufacturers who have conducted tests in accordance with ARI 350-86.

Therefore, it is recommended that the engineer specify noise limits in octave-band sound power levels from 125 Hz to 4000 Hz. These limits should be based on the room sound pressure level criterion assigned the receiving space, after conversion to sound power level.

Estimate the Maximum Allowable Sound Power

The designer can estimate and specify the maximum allowable sound power level in each octave band for a fan coil installation in a given room by using Equation 19 in Chapter 43 of the *1995 ASHRAE Handbook—HVAC Applications*.

NOISE SPECIFICATIONS

All room fan coil units listed in the schedule below shall have been tested in accordance with ARI Standard 350-86. When operating at the operating points shown, the values of sound power level (L_w) shall not exceed those scheduled in Table 12-2.

TABLE 12-2
Sample Room Fan Coil Unit Specification

Sound Specifications		Maximum L_w Values in dB *re* 1 Picowatt Octave-Band Center Frequency in Hz						
Mark	**Fan Speed**	**63**	**125**	**250**	**500**	**1k**	**2k**	**4k**
RFC-1	Low							
	Medium							
	High							

Chapter 13
Centrifugal Water Pumps

by *John Paulauskis and Warren Blazier*

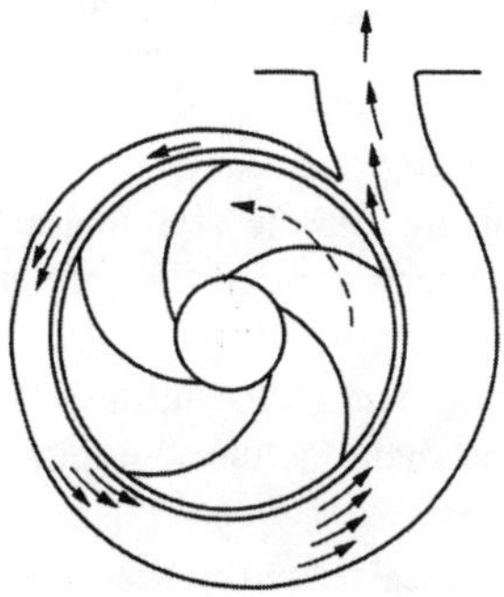

OVERVIEW

Centrifugal water pumps used in HVAC systems have a number of different physical configurations.[1] However, the acoustical characteristics are similar and can be grouped in terms of motor speed, volume flow rate, operating pressure, and impeller type.

Centrifugal pumps in HVAC systems are direct drive and operate at speeds of 1200 rpm, 1800 rpm, and 3600 rpm. The impeller blades typically number five and are backward curved in design. Therefore, the basic structure of a pump noise spectrum has two components: one that has a broad, continuous frequency distribution associated with the turbulent flow of the fluid, and one represented by a tonal component occurring at the blade passage rate (number of blades × the rpm/60 Hz). The tonal component typically

1. For an illustration of pump types, see Figure 1, Chapter 39 of *1992 ASHRAE Handbook—Systems and Equipment*.

occurs in the region of either 100 Hz, 150 Hz, or 300 Hz, depending on the motor rpm.

MANUFACTURERS' SOUND RATING PROCEDURES AND PRACTICES FOR CENTRIFUGAL WATER PUMPS

The availability of sound rating data from pump manufacturers is usually limited to averaged A-weighted sound pressure levels (dBA) measured at one meter from the pump. However, many manufacturers have no data available because pump noise is considered a system-related effect that is subject to many variables beyond the control of the pump manufacturer. A single pump size or type can be packaged with a variety of motor drives, be operated at several different speeds, have different impeller sizes, and be installed with many different pipe configurations.

The Hydraulic Institute is the organization most recognized as setting performance criteria for centrifugal water pumps. ANSI/HI 9.1-9.5 is a guideline established by the institute for the measurement of airborne sound level from pumps. However, this guideline does not require that manufacturers publish the measured data (ANSI/HI 1994).

ANSI/HI 9.1-9.5 1994 requires that octave-band sound pressure levels be measured at the eight octave mid-band frequencies between 63 Hz and 8000 Hz, in addition to the A-weighted sound level (dBA). The locations of the measurements are shown in Figure 13-1. Both location-specific and averaged sound data may be recorded and documented. Pump test conditions, including pump

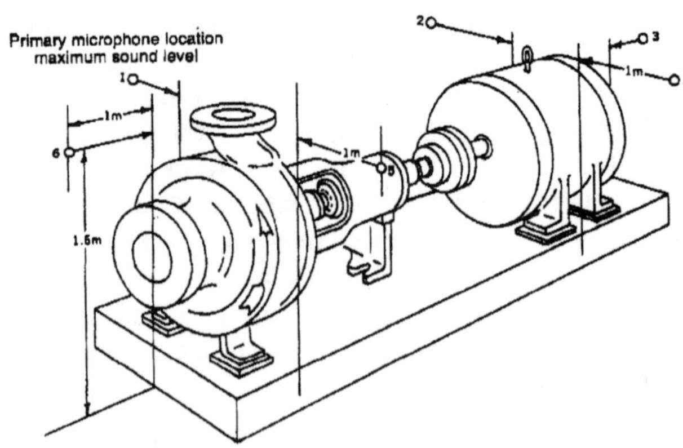

FIGURE 13-1 ANSI/HI 9.1-9.5 test configuration.

speed, capacity, and head pressure must be recorded, as well as the location of the pump in the test room and the level of ambient background sound.

It must be borne in mind that any pump noise data supplied by the manufacturer that is obtained from tests in accordance with ANSI/HI 9.1-9.5 includes both the noise of the drive motor and the radiated noise from piping and control valves installed within the test room. Thus, if the pump is supplied with a different motor, or installed in a different piping configuration, the submitted data may not be applicable.

UNCERTAINTIES IN SOUND RATING DATA

As with any laboratory test procedure, there are always measurement uncertainties to be taken into account when reporting data. Experience indicates that uncertainties in the probable accuracy of measurements, as shown in Table 13-1, should be considered when applying manufacturers' test data to an HVAC system design.

TABLE 13-1
Estimated Variability of Product Sound Pressure Data Due to Measurement Uncertainties and Production Quality Control
The Frequency Bands Most Affected by the Pump Load are Also Indicated by an x.

Centrifugal Water Pumps						
Octave Mid-Band Frequency Hz	**Measurement Uncertainty of ARI 575 Test Procedure[a] dB**	**Repeatability of Test Data[b] dB**	**Production Variability[c] dB**	**Cumulative Uncer-tainty Due To All Factors[d] dB**	**Variability of Random Sample *re* Catalog in Free Field[e] dB**	**Bands Most Affected by Pump Load dB**
63	± 3 dB	± 2 dB	± 4 dB	± 4 dB	+6, -0 dB	x
125	± 3 dB	± 1 dB	± 3 dB	± 3 dB	+5, -0 dB	x
250-500	± 2 dB	± 1 dB	± 3 dB	± 4 dB	+3, -0 dB	x
1000-4000	± 1.5 dB	± 1 dB	± 3 dB	± 4 dB	+3, -0 dB	
8000	± 2.5 dB	± 0.5 dB	± 3 dB	± 5 dB	+3, -0 dB	

a. Estimated standard deviation of includes variations due to different operators, measurement location, and instrumentation. (Based on data in ANSI Std. S12.10)
b. Repetitive testing of same unit in same laboratory.
c. Subject to manufacturing tolerances permitted in production quality control.
d. Based on the square root of the sum of the squares of all uncertainties.
e. Published catalog data are not customarily derived from a statistical sampling of production units but usually are determined by testing a prototype. Thus, the results of testing random production samples would tend to exceed those published by the manufacturer.

APPLICATION OF CENTRIFUGAL PUMP SOUND RATINGS TO BUILDING SYSTEMS

Pump noise problems usually occur in locations remote to the actual installation. The disturbance is typically associated with a tonal component at the pump blade-passage frequency, which is perceived as a hum or whine. The path along which this component of pump noise reaches a remote location is complex in that it may be fluidborne, structureborne, or a combination of the two. The end result is that noise is radiated to the surrounding area by the pipe wall. If the pipe is allowed to make physical contact with a building surface at a wall or floor penetration, the resulting airborne noise radiation, due to the structural excitation of the extended surfaces, can be substantial.

Data obtained in accordance with the ANSI/HI guidelines only pertains to the noise emitted by the pump and drive motor. It does not consider any effects due to pipe-wall radiated noise outside the test room. Thus, manufacturers' sound data is only applicable to the mechanical space in which the pump is installed.

RECOMMENDED DESIGN AND INSTALLATION PRACTICES FOR CENTRIFUGAL WATER PUMPS

A significant noise reduction at the pump blade-passage frequency can usually be obtained by trimming the impeller tips to approximately 80% of maximum diameter. This can usually be accomplished with only a minor reduction in pump performance. However, this noise control solution is not recommended for systems that are already marginal with respect to pump capacity.

In principal, the pump noise problems that occur at remote locations from the pump can be avoided by ensuring that the piping is carried on isolation hangers, resiliently sleeved at wall and floor penetrations, and supported on isolation mounts at anchor points. In reality, these precautions do not always function as intended because the resiliently supported piping is free to undergo unrestrained movements induced by changing hydraulic thrust forces within the system. Problems of this nature are prone to occur when the piping is carried on resilient hangers, and the layout of the piping system must be studied to determine where it is advisable to install anchors or thrust restraints.

The typical resilient pipe hanger is comprised of a neoprene or spring isolator that supports the piping load through a rod that passes through a clearance opening in the bottom of the hanger body. Isolation occurs as long as the connecting rod does not make physical contact with the clearance opening in the hanger body. However, a simple action, such as the hydraulic shock produced by the starting or stopping of a pump, can result in sufficient piping movement to short-circuit the hanger rod to the hanger body and negate the isolation. Unfortunately, because so many variables are involved, it is difficult to determine in advance the nature of these piping movements and where in the system short circuiting is likely to occur. The best precaution is to select a resilient hanger with a design that can accommodate sufficient lateral movement to minimize the potential for short circuiting. Typical hangers of this type are available that usually permit angular misalignments of ±15° to occur without short circuiting.

Pump noise transmitted to remote locations can be significantly reduced by attenuating components of fluidborne noise as close to the pump as practical and by introducing a break in the structureborne noise path. One method of control is to use energy-absorbing neoprene couplings, such as illustrated in Figure 13-2, in the piping connections to both the suction and discharge sides of the pump. The spherical cross section of the design allows the coupling to uniformly expand and contract in response to the fluctuating pressure pulses at the blade passing frequency. The noise attenuation achieved using this method is claimed to be 10 dB or greater.[2] However, this type of spherical connector should not be confused with steel bellows type connectors, which offer stress relief due to pipe misalignment but do not provide noise reduction.

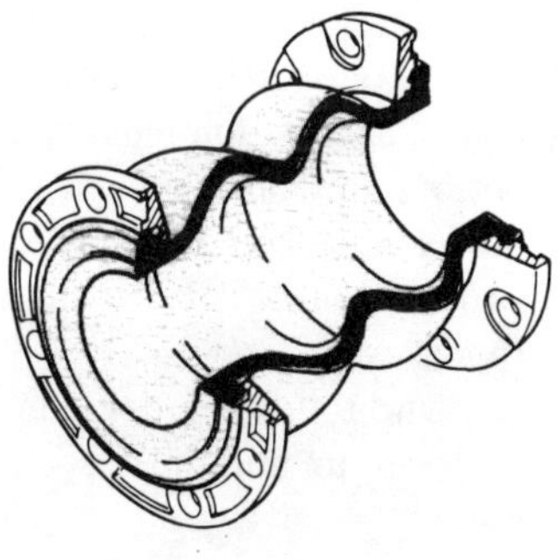

FIGURE 13-2 Twin sphere in-line connector.

Caution should be observed when using neoprene flexible couplings in hot water systems. One of the authors has experienced degradation and fatigue of neoprene couplings as temperatures approached within 20°F of the manufacturer's published upper limit in hot water applications.

2. Field test data from Mason Industries, Inc.

SUGGESTED NOISE AND VIBRATION ISOLATION SPECIFICATIONS

VIBRATION ISOLATION OF PUMP ASSEMBLY

The reader is referred to Table 42 in Chapter 43 of the *1995 ASHRAE Handbook—Applications* and subsequent handbook revisions for recommendations concerning the vibration isolation of centrifugal water pumps.

NOISE SPECIFICATIONS

There are industry guidelines published by the Hydraulic Institute for specifying the sound pressure levels of centrifugal pumps. However, these will only identify the airborne noise radiated from the pump/motor assembly within the mechanical equipment room. Therefore, it is important to specify the pump installation requirements, such as the method of isolation between the pump and supporting structure, as well as the type of flexible couplings in the piping and their location to reduce the transmission of fluid and structureborne noise to areas outside the mechanical equipment room.

The following five-part specification should assist the design engineer to minimize noise problems from all aspects of pump noise.

1. The centrifugal water pump(s) shall be tested at design conditions in accordance with ANSI/HI 9.1-9.5. The average sound pressure levels in the eight octave bands between 63 Hz and 8000 Hz shall not exceed the levels shown in Table 13-2.
2. Piping attached to the pump shall be isolated with single (or twin) sphere neoprene flexible pipe connectors on both the suction and discharge sides of the pump(s). Neoprene/rubber connectors shall not be utilized when water temperatures are within 20°F of manufacturers' published high temperature limit.
3. Piping within 100 ft of the pump(s) shall be isolated from all structural elements that can transmit noise to an occupied space. Isolation shall consist of spring (or neoprene) isolation hangers for suspended piping, and isolation sleeves shall be used where pipes penetrate walls and floors. Isolation hangers shall be adjusted so that hanger

rods do not come into contact with the isolator housing where the rod passes through the housing.

4. The centrifugal pump shall be securely anchored to the support base and in combination with the vibration isolation as scheduled on the drawings.
5. The centrifugal pump shall be realigned with motor, couplings, and all connected piping after installation. Alignment shall be made so that no undo stress is applied to the equipment, connected piping, or structure. Noise shall not be transmitted to any support structure, connected surface, or adjacent environment.

TABLE 13-2

Maximum Sound Pressure Levels for Centrifugal Pumps, dB[a]

	Octave-Band Center Frequency in Hz							
Mark	**63**	**125**	**250**	**500**	**1k**	**2k**	**4k**	**8k**
P-1								
P-2								

a. Measurements conducted in accordance with ANSI/HI 9.1-9.5.

REFERENCES

ANSI/HI. 1994. *ANSI/HI 9.1-9.5 1994, Pumps—General guidelines.* New York: American National Standards Institute. Hydraulic Institute.

Chapter 14
Air-Cooled Chillers and Condensing Units

by *Warren Blazier*

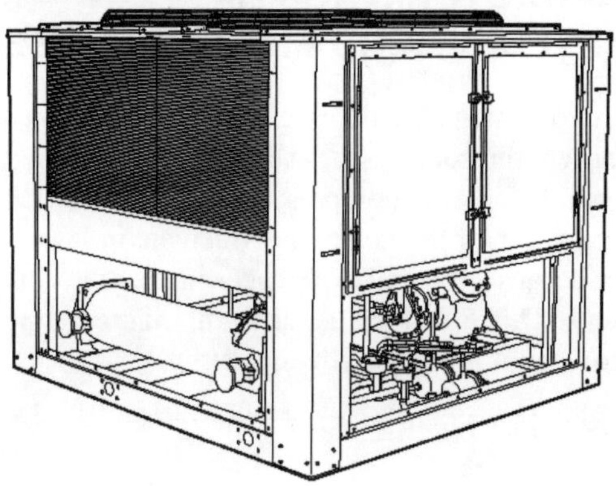

OVERVIEW

Air-cooled water chillers are used in industrial and commercial applications and range in size from about 50 tons to 450 tons. Air-cooled condensing units are used in somewhat smaller capacity applications in conjunction with an indoor direct-expansion evaporator package. In residential applications, for example, product sizes range from 1 ton to 12 tons. Commercial applications of air-cooled condensing units usually do not exceed 75 tons. Air-cooled chillers and condensing units are installed outdoors so that the heat of compression in the refrigeration cycle can be rejected by the action of induced-draft propeller fans, which draw outside air across the condenser coil(s).

The air-cooled chiller has a lower first-cost than a water-cooled chiller because a separate cooling tower and associated water piping is not required in the heat rejection portion of the cycle. However, the operating noise level of an air-cooled chiller is significantly higher than the equivalent water-cooled chiller because of the increased noise resulting from the addition of condenser fans and the wide use of semihermetic compressors. Also, the fact that these units are installed outdoors rather than indoors makes them highly vulnerable to complaints from the surrounding neighborhood. In general, the overall level of fan noise produced by an air-cooled chiller is much higher than that of the cooling tower fans in an equivalent water-cooled system. The reason is that a substantially greater quantity of air is required, on a cfm/ton basis, to offset the fact that there is no evaporative cooling.

NOISE CHARACTERISTICS OF AIR-COOLED CHILLERS AND CONDENSERS

The two principal sources of noise in air-cooled chillers and condensers are the compressor and the condenser fan. In addition, if a unit contains multiple compressors and condenser fans, the time-amplitude pattern of the noise may fluctuate in level due to "beats" that occur because of small differences in the motor speed of similar components. This effect can significantly increase the potential for a noise complaint in a borderline situation.

COMPRESSOR NOISE

The semihermetic reciprocating and the rotary screw are two types of compressors normally used in air-cooled chillers. Of the two, the screw compressor is substantially noisier when compared on the basis of equal capacity. Such a comparison is illustrated in Figure 14-1 for nominal 100 ton reciprocating and screw compressor units.[1] In this example, it will be noted that the octave-band sound power level spectrum of the generic screw compressor is nominally flat, whereas that of the semihermetic reciprocating compressor is "haystack" in shape, peaking in the region of 500 Hz. A more detailed analysis of these spectra, such as in one-third octave bands, will reveal that the structure is a series of discrete-frequency (tonal) components for both compressor types. In the case of the reciprocating unit, the components appear at the shaft frequency

1. Data for the reciprocating compressor were drawn from Chapter 42 of the *1991 ASHRAE Handbook—Applications*. Data for the screw compressor are a composite of manufacturers' published data.

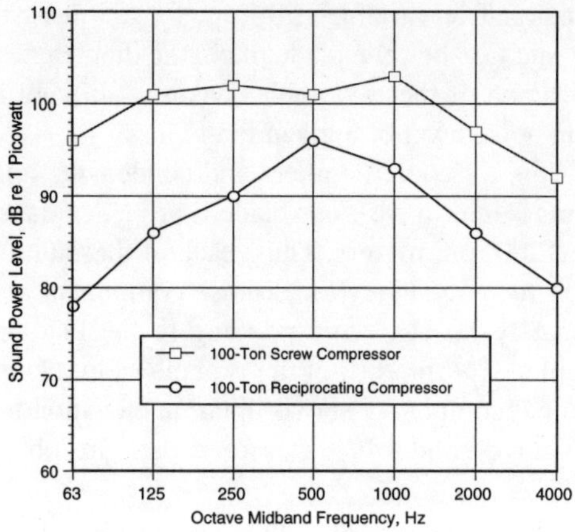

FIGURE 14-1 Comparison of sound power level spectra: Nominal 100-ton, screw vs. reciprocating compressor.

(rpm/60) and at a series of harmonics of shaft speed × the number of pistons/60. The screw compressor produces strong components at the shaft speed/60 and at a series of harmonics of the shaft speed × the number of lobes/60.

The human ear is less tolerant of audible compressor noise (because of the discrete-frequency character of the spectra) than the relatively broad-band character of the condenser fan noise. Thus, the level of compressor noise from an air-cooled chiller is frequently more a factor in invoking neighborhood complaints than the broad-band noise associated with the condenser fans. The exception to this rule is when the tonal blade passage frequency of the condenser fans reaches a level of 65 dB to 70 dB or higher at the receiver location. In multi-fan units, the fact that the motors turn at slightly different speeds causes beats in the time-pattern of blade-frequency noise, which is annoying to the ear.

Condenser Fan Noise

The condenser fans in air-cooled water chillers and condensing units are of the propeller type and draw outside air across the condenser coil(s) to reject the heat of compression in the refrigeration cycle. The number of fans utilized depends upon the configuration of the condenser coils and the rated total capacity of the unit.

There is significant variation among manufacturers in the number and physical design of propeller fans used in chiller equipment of similar capacity. For this reason, there is also a large variation in the level of condenser fan noise associated with competitive units of similar capacity. The variables in propeller fan design include the blade shape and number, the blade pitch, the diameter, and the operating speed. Each of these variables has a significant influence on the operating noise level of a given fan type.

Most of the air-cooled chillers and condensing units presently being manufactured have four-bladed propeller fans driven by direct-drive 1200 rpm motors. Thus, each of these units produces a characteristic low-frequency tonal noise component at a frequency of approximately 80 Hz, corresponding to the blade-passage rate (number of blades × rpm/60) of the propeller fan. (The presence of this 80 Hz tonal component shows up as an elevation in the level of the 63 Hz octave band when measured data are obtained on this basis.)

Figure 14-2 shows the difficulty of detecting the presence of this blade-frequency component with only octave-band data in comparison to the more revealing one-third octave-band analysis. It is the presence of this blade-passage frequency component that is one of the more common causes for neighborhood complaints because the human ear is significantly less tolerant of noise of tonal character than it is of the broad-band noise of the remainder of the propeller fan spectrum.

Because of differences in design configuration and choices of propeller fan type, the level of the 80 Hz blade-frequency compo-

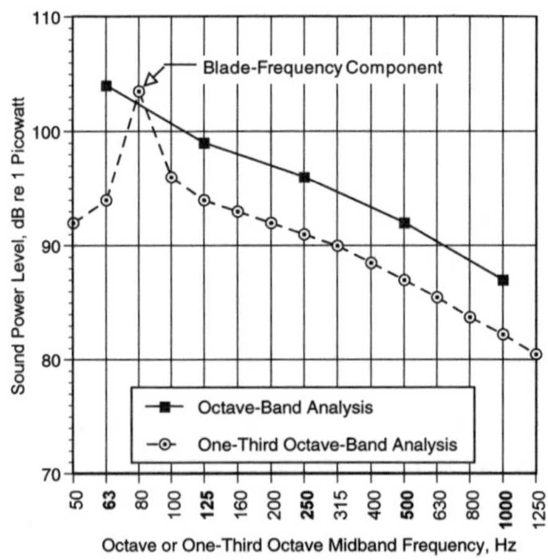

FIGURE 14-2 Comparison between octave-band and one-third octave-band analyses in detecting a blade-passage frequency component at 80 Hz, present in the noise spectrum of a four-bladed propeller fan operating at 1200 rpm.

nent can vary by as much as 10 dB in units of the same capacity presently available from different manufacturers. This can represent the difference between a complaint and a noncomplaint situation in a given installation. An additional problem arises from the beats that occur because of the slip in the motor rpm with load. Each propeller may be running at a slightly different rpm, resulting in significant irritating time-modulation caused by the multiple beats between each fan and its adjacent counterpart.

COMPOSITE OF CONDENSER FAN PLUS COMPRESSOR NOISE

The level of condenser fan noise in currently marketed chiller equipment, while variable from manufacturer to manufacturer, tends to show similar trends as a function of chiller capacity. However, the largest variable from unit to unit is in the level of compressor noise, which is a function of the type of compressor used. Presently, chillers using screw compressors are substantially noisier than those using reciprocating equipment.

AIR-COOLED CHILLERS AND CONDENSING UNITS USING RECIPROCATING COMPRESSORS

Figure 14-3 illustrates the composite sound power level spectrum of a nominal air-cooled 100-ton chiller containing reciprocat-

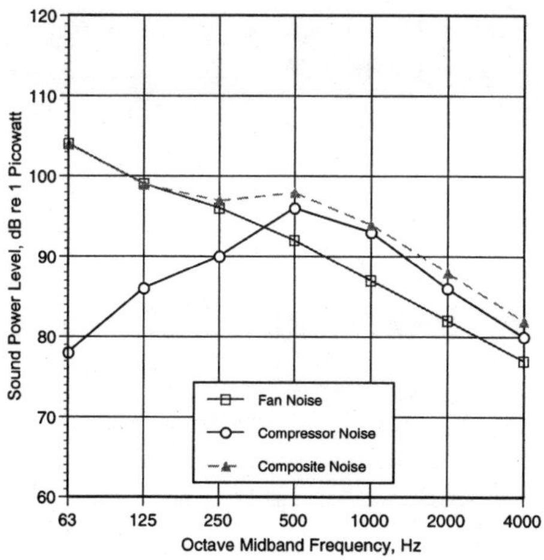

FIGURE 14-3 Composite sound power level spectrum of a typical 100-ton air-cooled chiller using reciprocating compressors.

ing compressors. In this example, it can be seen that the fan noise dominates the composite spectrum in the frequency region below 500 Hz. In the spectrum at 500 Hz and above, the compressor noise is higher by about 4 dB on the average. This relationship between the relative levels of compressor and condenser fan noise tends to not vary significantly with the size of the unit since both component noise levels are nominally directly proportional to capacity.

AIR-COOLED CHILLERS USING SCREW COMPRESSORS

Figure 14-4 illustrates the composite sound power level spectrum of a nominal 100-ton air-cooled chiller containing screw compressors. In this example, it can be seen that the noise of the screw compressor substantially exceeds that of the condenser fans in the frequency range above 125 Hz. In fact, the magnitude by which the level of the compressor noise spectrum exceeds that of the fan is about 12 dB on the average! Therefore, if the noise level associated with the use of a chiller containing screw compressors is compared to one using reciprocating equipment (previous example), it is clear that the additional noise control requirements to meet a specified objective are at least 8 dB or greater. This is a very significant difference. In terms of relative loudness, as judged by the human ear, the screw chiller is about twice as loud as a reciprocating chiller. In terms of the relative cost of introducing 8 dB more noise control, the difference is substantial.

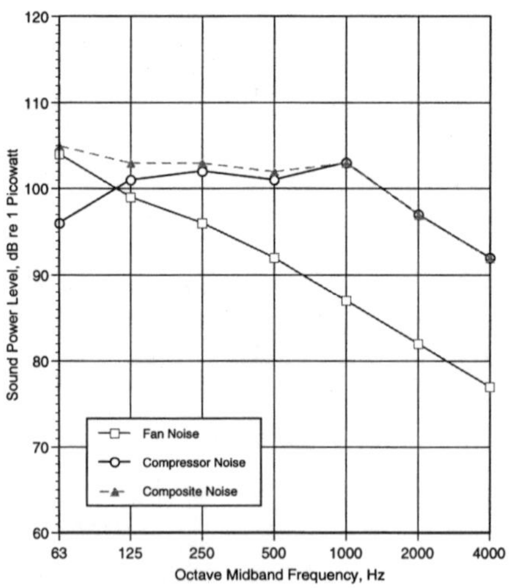

FIGURE 14-4 The composite sound power level spectrum of a typical 100-ton air-cooled chiller using screw compressors.

SOUND STANDARDS AND DATA AVAILABILITY

LARGE AIR-COOLED CHILLER AND CONDENSING UNITS

The Air-Conditioning and Refrigeration Institute (ARI) is the cognizant industry trade association for the development of sound rating standards for large air-cooled chiller and condensing units. At the present time, the applicable rating standard is *ARI-370-86, Sound Rating of Large Outdoor Refrigerating and Air-Conditioning Equipment.* ARI Standard 370-86 specifies procedures for determining the sound power level of the equipment operating at ARI standard thermal rating conditions. These data are processed to yield the standard sound rating. Tests conducted at other than specified operating conditions are identified as application sound ratings. The test environment may be either outdoors, where tests are conducted under free-field conditions, or inside a reverberant room, anechoic, or hemianechoic facility equipped to load the unit at the specified operating point(s). In general, manufacturers test outdoors under free-field conditions in order to avoid the high cost of constructing an indoor test environment of a size large enough to accommodate their line of equipment, including integral facilities for thermal loading.

The acoustical data resulting from the use of ARI-370-86 are expressed in terms of octave-band sound power levels, which have been determined in accordance with the appropriate procedure specified by ANSI for the test environment utilized. The raw data are in the form of octave-band sound power levels over the recommended frequency range from 63 Hz to 8000 Hz. These data are processed by A-weighting the individual octave-band levels and logarithmically summing the weighted values to yield a single number, the A-weighted sound power level. The A-weighted sound power level is expressed in bels to avoid confusion with the A-weighted sound pressure level, which is expressed in decibels. (One bel is equal to ten decibels.) The sound rating obtained in accordance with ARI-370-86 is the A-weighted sound power level, $L_w(A)$, expressed in bels. In addition, the unweighted octave-band sound power levels are also available for noise control purposes in the design of shielding barriers.[2]

---

2. Unfortunately, Standard 370 specifies that measurements below the 125 Hz octave band are optional. Therefore, data corresponding to the prominent blade-passage frequency of the condenser fan, which is nearly always present (see Figure 14-2), may not be available.

Air-Cooled Condensing Units Less than 12 Tons

ARI Standard 270-84, Sound Rating of Outdoor Unitary Equipment, is applicable for sound rating air-cooled condensing units 12 tons and lower. The measured test data utilized in developing the rating are expressed as one-third octave-band sound power levels over the frequency range from 100 Hz to 10,000 Hz.

The first step in arriving at a sound rating is to apply adjustments to the measured data to account for any discrete frequency (tonal) components that may be present, using a detailed procedure specified in the standard.[3] The second step is to apply A-weighted corrections to the adjusted one-third octave-band data and to logarithmically sum the result to yield the ARI sound rating, SR_{ARI}. The SR_{ARI} is identified as the tone-corrected A-weighted sound power level, expressed in bels.

APPLICATION OF SOUND RATING DATA TO FIELD INSTALLATIONS

Air-Cooled Chillers

The $L_w(A)$, determined in accordance with ARI Standard 370, is principally of value in establishing the potential for compliance with a community noise ordinance or other regulations that are frequently expressed in terms of A-weighted sound pressure levels, $L_p(A)$, at an adjacent property line. It must be recognized that these are two different metrics (power level vs. pressure level) and that a conversion is required before a comparison can be made.[4]

Beyond the application to community noise ordinances, the $L_w(A)$ ARI standard sound rating is of little value. If after application of the appropriate correction factor for source to receiver distance it is found that the specified limit will be exceeded, the

3. In an earlier version of the methodology (ARI 270-67), this tone-correction procedure was coupled with a second procedure to assign rating penalties for tonal content and an adverse spectrum shape. However, this companion second procedure is not incorporated in the current ARI Standard 270-84, thus making the basis for the tone-correction step meaningless.
4. Refer to Chapter 2 of this book for a discussion of the relationship between sound power level and pressure level and to Chapter 43 of the *1995 ASHRAE Handbook—Applications* for guidance in choosing the appropriate conversion factors.

octave-band sound power level data based on measurements in accordance with ARI Standard 370 will be required in order to engineer suitable noise control measures. Should one elect to design a barrier to shield the noise source from the receiver (this is usually the only practical option with air-cooled chillers), the availability of octave-band acoustical data is essential. For a discussion of barrier design principles, see Chapter 43 of the *1995 ASHRAE Handbook—Applications*.

AIR-COOLED CONDENSING UNITS LESS THAN 12 TONS

ARI Standard 275-84, Application of Sound Rated Outdoor Unitary Equipment, is an application standard that may be used to estimate the A-weighted sound level at a chosen location, such as a neighboring property line, using the SR_{ARI} sound power level rating of a product tested in accordance with ARI Standard 270-84. ARI 275-84 also prescribes a procedure for estimating the noise reduction performance of a barrier installed in the path between the source and receiver. However, the reliability of this procedure is questionable because the barrier performance depends upon the spectrum characteristics of the noise source, and these must be estimated if only the A-weighted rating is used.

UNCERTAINTIES IN THE APPLICATION OF MANUFACTURERS' DATA

There are several factors that can affect the reliability of manufacturers' data. Table 14-1 lists uncertainties that should be recognized in field application of the data.

RECOMMENDED DESIGN AND INSTALLATION PRACTICES

While there are a number of designs a manufacturer can produce to minimize noise, the system designer and/or installer of the equipment in the application has only a few options to consider. Obviously, if there are several potential locations for the equipment, the best choice is a location farthest away from neighboring property or a location where natural shielding exists because of adjacent structures or roof parapets. If, on the other hand, the only available location has direct line-of-sight to a sensitive receiver, the construction of a barrier wall is about the only viable noise control solution. It should be borne in mind that nighttime ambient sound levels are

TABLE 14-1
Estimated Variability of Product Sound Power Data Due to Measurement Uncertainties and Production Quality Control

Air-Cooled Chillers and Condensing Units					
Octave Mid-Band Frequency Hz	Measurement Uncertainty of Std. Test Procedure[a] dB	Repeatability of Test Data[b] dB	Production Variability[c] dB	Cumulative Uncertainty Due to All Previous Factors[d] dB	Variability of Random Sample *re* Catalog[e] dB
63	± 4	± 2	± 4	± 6	+6, -0
125	± 3	± 1	± 3	±4	+5, -0
250	± 2	± 1	± 3	± 4	+3, -0
500-4000	± 1.5	± 1	± 3	± 4	+3, -0
8000	± 3	± 0.5	± 3	± 4	+3, -0

a. Standard deviation of octave-band data per ISO 3741.
b. Repetitive testing of same unit in same laboratory.
c. Subject to manufacturing tolerances permitted in production quality control.
d. Based on the square root of the sum of the squares of all uncertainties.
e. Published catalog data are not customarily derived from a statistical sampling of production units but usually are determined by testing a prototype. Thus, the results of testing random production samples would tend to exceed those published by the manufacturer.

usually much lower than daytime levels. Therefore, if the equipment is to be operated at night, it is advisable to take into account the level of the prevailing nighttime ambient when designing the barrier.

BARRIER SOUND ATTENUATION

The acoustical efficiency of a barrier depends upon the difference in path length between the direct line-of-sight distance from source to receiver and the path over the barrier. As the difference in path length approaches zero (just breaks the line-of-sight), the attenuation provided by a barrier is limited to 5 dB or less. However, as the height of the barrier is increased to increase the difference in path length, the resulting noise reduction at the receiver location increases rapidly up to a practical limit of about 15 dB to 17 dB. One limitation to be aware of in optimizing a barrier design is the need to allow adequate space for the air to enter the condenser coil unrestricted. The recommendations of the manufacturer with respect to the minimum free space between the condenser coil(s) and the barrier should always be followed.

A mistake frequently made in the design of barriers for air-cooled chiller and condenser equipment is to assume that the location of the source is at the geometric center of the equipment, as viewed in elevation. This is incorrect for typical air-cooled equipment. The location of the fan noise source is at the top of the unit, and a conservative designer should consider the closest chiller surface to the property line in plan view. While it might be thought that the source of compressor noise is lower in elevation, this is not generally the case because the condenser coils located near the top of the unit are connected to the compressor through the refrigerant circuit and, thus, radiate a significant fraction of this component noise. Therefore, if the geometric center of the equipment is taken as the source location, the effective barrier height can be several feet less than assumed in the calculations, and the barrier performance measured in the field may prove to be significantly less than calculated.

Compressor Jacketing or Enclosure

The acoustical jacketing of compressors[5] can reduce their radiated noise by 10 dB to 15 dB at 500 Hz to 4000 Hz, depending upon the quality of the installation. A good quality jacketing system will include a soft decoupling layer of fiberglass applied to the compressor housing, surrounded by a weatherproof outer jacket that is structurally isolated from the body of the compressor. This outer jacket should consist of a "limp" material, such as barium-loaded vinyl, weighing at least 1 lb. per square foot of surface. Piping that is directly connected to the compressor should receive a similar treatment within the compressor compartment. It is also advisable to vibration isolate the compressor from the unit frame to avoid flanking by structureborne noise.

Enclosures around compressors require careful design so as to not create undamped flat metal surfaces that can re-radiate acoustically coupled compressor noise. Sheetmetal panel enclosures are capable of reducing compressor noise by 10 dB to 20 dB at all frequencies if the panels are at least 18 ga sheet steel, reinforced in both directions on 18 in. centers, and insulated inside with minimum 1 in. thick fiberglass. However, the compressor must be vibration isolated from the unit frame and the panels structurally

5. Compressor jacketing cannot prevent stuctureborne noise that is transmitted from the compressor to the condenser coils or to other chiller surfaces from radiating. Hence, compressor jacketing will only be effective when the compressor surface is the major radiator of compressor noise.

decoupled from the compressor, using resilient gasketing or seals, for the enclosure to be acoustically effective. Furthermore, whenever designing a compressor enclosure, it is important to make certain that the size and location of the enclosure will not significantly affect the entering airflow pattern to the condenser coils.

Noise Reduction at Night by System Operational Control Sequence

Large air-cooled chillers, containing multiple compressors and condenser fans, tend to operate at reduced noise levels under part-load conditions because the controls are typically sequenced to deactivate components not required to meet the demand. However, the extent to which noise levels can be reduced depends upon how the unit is actually configured to respond to changes in load.

In the case of air-cooled chillers using screw compressors where the compressor noise dominates that of the fans, if the load is matched by simply reducing the number of operating compressors and condenser fans, the noise levels at 50% or 25% of full capacity should be 3 dB or 6 dB lower, respectively, in all octave bands. On the other hand, with reciprocating compressor chiller equipment where the predominant noise is produced by the condenser fans, reducing the operating speed of the fans, as a part of the system control sequence, is potentially capable of significantly reducing noise. For example, shutting down one-half of the fans to meet 50% of design load represents a noise reduction of only 3 dB, whereas operating all the fans at one-half the speed can result in a 10 dB to 15 dB noise reduction. However, the compressor spectrum may then likely dominate and require jacketing or enclosure of the compressor body to preserve the effectiveness of the fan noise reduction. As control systems become more sophisticated, modulating fan speed will likely receive greater consideration in minimizing the part-load noise level of air-cooled chillers.

VIBRATION ISOLATION CONSIDERATIONS

When air-cooled chillers or condensing units are installed outdoors on a grade-slab, there is rarely a need to consider vibration isolation. A possible exception is with equipment installed adjacent to laboratory or production facilities that are extremely sensitive to groundborne vibration. In these cases, the advice of a consultant should be sought to ascertain the specific requirements for vibration isolation.

For air-cooled equipment installed in rooftop locations, the use of combination spring and neoprene vibration isolators in mounting compressors and flexible connectors in the attached refrigerant piping is strongly recommended.[6]

SUGGESTED NOISE SPECIFICATIONS

Specifications for air-cooled chiller equipment, destined for a given application, must take into account at least the following factors:

1. Site plan: location of nearest noise-sensitive neighbor or the closest property line at which community noise may be an issue. It is also advisable to determine what the daytime/nighttime background noise levels are in the neighborhood of the installation.
2. The most likely location of the equipment on the site, and the distance to the nearest noise-sensitive neighbor or property line.
3. Feasibility of constructing a barrier of practical height as a noise control measure.

On the basis of (1) and (2) above, it is possible to specify the equipment sound power level that will not exceed the noise limit at the property line by using the procedure described in ARI Standard 275-84 to determine the appropriate power level/pressure level conversion factor. If this is done, the engineer need only specify the maximum A-weighted sound power level, $L_w(A)$, determined in accordance with ARI Standard 370-86. (Since the ARI sound rating, SR_{ARI}, is expressed in bels, it will be necessary to convert this rating number to decibels by multiplying by 10).

Should it be found that no equipment is available that meets the requirement specified above, then either a barrier design must be considered or the equipment location must be changed to increase the source to receiver distance. If the equipment cannot be relocated and it is determined that a barrier is required, the manufacturer should provide octave-band sound power level data to facilitate an appropriate barrier design whose noise attenuation is equivalent to the difference between the equipment sound rating and the calculated requirement.

---

6. For general guidelines, refer to Table 42 and footnotes appearing in Chapter 43 of the *1995 ASHRAE Handbook—Applications*.

NOISE SPECIFICATIONS

All air-cooled water chillers listed in the schedule below shall have been tested in accordance with ARI-370-86, Sound Rating of Large Outdoor Refrigerating and Air-Conditioning Equipment. *When operating at the operating points shown, the values of sound power level* (L_W) *shall not exceed those scheduled in Table 14-2.*

TABLE 14-2
Sample Air-Cooled Water Chiller Specification

Sound Specifications								
Mark	**dBA**	**63**	**125**	**250**	**500**	**1k**	**2k**	**4k**
ACC-1								

Chapter 15
Water-Cooled Chillers

by *Charles Ebbing and Warren Blazier*

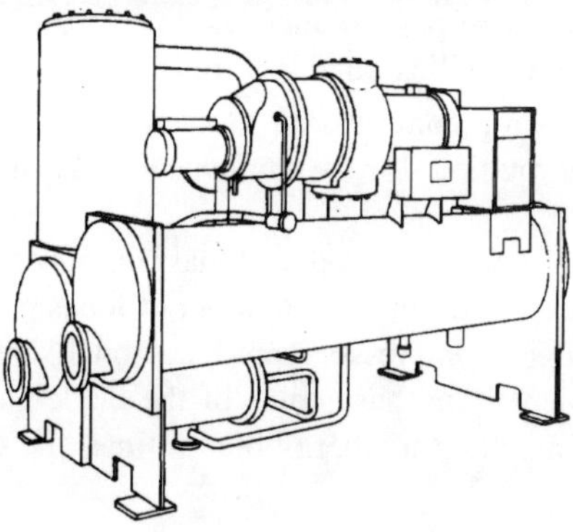

OVERVIEW

Table 15-1 shows the types and typical tonnage ranges for water-cooled chillers presently available in the marketplace. These units use either the absorption heat transfer process or compressors coupled to condensers and evaporators to produce chilled water or brine for delivery to a remote cooling coil(s) located in air handlers or room terminals.

TABLE 15-1
Chiller Tonnage Range

Chiller Type	Typical Size Range in Tons
Absorption	10 to 2000 tons
Reciprocating	15 to 300 tons
Screw	15 to 600 tons
Centrifugal	100 to 10,000+ tons

While absorption chillers produce little noise of concern, the noise from reciprocating, screw, or centrifugal compressors can cause problems, particularly when installed in the vicinity of noise sensitive areas.

Water-cooled condensing units can be installed either indoors or outdoors since the building heat rejection by the condenser is usually transferred to a cooling tower connected to a local water source. The noise produced by water-cooled chillers is a function of the cooling capacity, compressor head pressure, and flow-volume of the refrigerant, as well as the type of the compression technology utilized. Reciprocating, centrifugal, and screw-type chillers produce a combination of both broad-band and multiple tonal components. Significant tonal components typically occur at multiples of the blade, piston, or lobe-pass frequency.

For example, as illustrated in Table 15-2,

- reciprocating compressors produce tonal frequency components at multiples of the shaft speed times the number of pistons;
- screw compressors produce tonal components at multiples of the shaft speed times the number of lobes;
- centrifugal compressors produce tonal components at the fundamental and harmonics of the blade-passage frequency of the impeller (number of blades times the shaft speed).

NOISE CHARACTERISTICS OF WATER-COOLED CHILLERS

Sound data for water-cooled chillers are based on the measurement of sound pressure levels and are usually measured in a *free*

TABLE 15-2
Tonal Components of Chiller Types and the Frequency Range in Which they Typically Occur

Type of Water Chiller	Octave Band Range Containing Tones	Tone Mechanism (Hz)
Reciprocating Chiller	125-2000 Hz	(rpm)×(# pistons)/60 plus harmonics
Screw Chiller	250-1000 Hz	(rpm)×(# lobes)/60 plus harmonics
Centrifugal Chiller	1000-8000 Hz	(rpm)×(# impeller blades)/ 60 plus harmonics

field[1] at a distance of one meter from the chiller rather than in terms of sound power level, as is the convention in rating most other HVAC components. The reason for this is that water chillers, like cooling towers, are often too large in physical size to be evaluated in most acoustical test facilities. Furthermore, for the tests to be meaningful, the machinery must be tested at a loaded condition, which is generally beyond the capabilities of most acoustical facilities. For this reason, it is important to understand the differences between sound pressure and sound power in interpreting the noise ratings of chiller equipment. The differences between sound pressure and sound power are discussed in Chapter 2.

MANUFACTURERS' SOUND RATING PROCEDURES AND PRACTICES FOR WATER-COOLED CHILLERS

COGNIZANT INDUSTRY TRADE ASSOCIATION

The Air-Conditioning and Refrigeration Institute (ARI) develops the standards for noise measurement of chiller equipment. The standard applicable to the sound measurement of water-cooled chillers (which are generally installed indoors) is *ARI 575-95, Method of Measuring Machinery Sound Within an Equipment Space*.

SOUND MEASUREMENTS PER ARI-575-95

ARI-575-95 specifies the method for noise measurement of water-cooled chiller equipment. However, unlike most other ARI standards, ARI-575-95 is not a rating standard because the acoustical characteristics of the test environment are not specified. In spite of this, the HVAC industry uses this standard as the basis for publishing chiller noise ratings.

It generally is not practical to determine the sound *power* level of large equipment such as water-cooled chillers in most industry acoustical test facilities presently available because this requires the use of huge reverberant test rooms with facilities for thermodynamic loading of the equipment that would be prohibitively expensive. As an alternative, ARI-575 specifies a method of measuring close-in sound *pressure* levels in an operating installation. Such data are of value in assessing the need for wearing hearing protec-

1. Measurements are often made in spaces that approach outdoor free-field conditions.

tion devices when working in the vicinity of the equipment or for estimating the sound transmission loss requirements for isolating the chiller noise from adjacent occupied spaces.

ARI 575-95 specifies a procedure that requires the measurement of sound pressure levels at a series of prescribed locations at a height of 1.5 m above the floor and at 1 m from the surface of the equipment. Other than prohibiting measurements close to nearby reflective surfaces, ARI 575-95 does not specify the acoustical environment in which the equipment is to be installed for test. Consequently, the reported or measured sound pressure levels at 1 m from the surface of the equipment will vary as a function of both the physical size of the test room and the amount of acoustical absorption present in the space; the larger the test room, or the more acoustically absorbent the environment, the *lower* the measured sound pressure levels will be. As a rule, most manufacturers conduct measurements in large factory spaces or in an essentially free-field, nonreflective environment, such as outdoors. Thus, published sound pressure level rating data that are obtained under these conditions most likely will be significantly lower than those measured in typical mechanical rooms in field installations of the equipment.[2]

ARI 575-95 specifies the measurement of sound pressure levels at 1 m intervals around the equipment on a grid 1 m from an imaginary box that will just fit over the machine, as illustrated in Figure 15-1.

Figure 15-2 shows a typical grid and the points at which the measurements of sound pressure level are to be made. The A-weighted sound level (dBA) is recorded at each measurement location, and octave-band sound pressure levels are measured at four "key" points. The sound rating of the

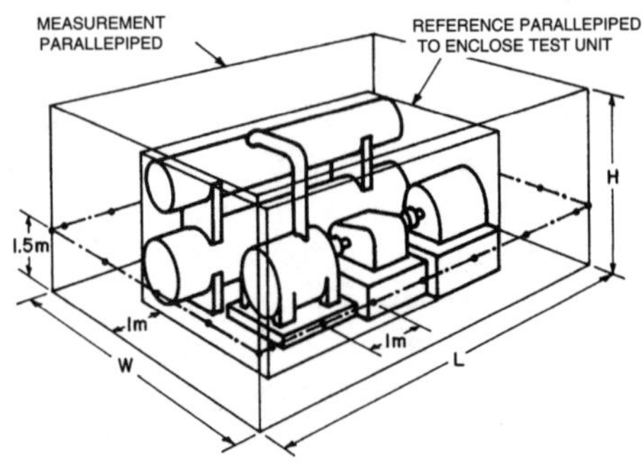

FIGURE 15-1 ARI 575-95 measurement geometry.

2. Newly revised refrigerant equipment safety standards, such as *ASHRAE Standard 15-1994, Safety Code for Mechanical Refrigeration*, has promulgated the use of small individual mechanical equipment rooms for water-cooled chillers.

unit is the logarithmic average of the A-weighted sound levels (dBA) obtained at all specified measurement locations. The octave-band data obtained at the four key points are likewise averaged on a logarithmic basis to provide spectrum information. ARI 575-95 also specifies a procedure for spatial averaging at the measurement locations if a standing wave is detected.

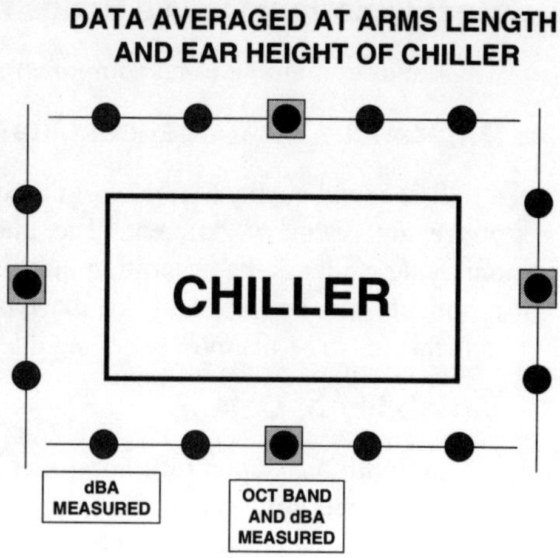

FIGURE 15-2 ARI 575-95 measurement grid.

OVERVIEW OF ARI 575 TEST PROCEDURE

Noise Sources Measured by Standard ARI-575

The measurement of chiller noise in accordance with ARI-575-95 is a composite of all noise sources radiating from the equipment surfaces, including the existing ambient noise. For both centrifugal and screw chillers, the noise levels are usually highest close to the discharge line and condenser shell. The sound data available from tests conducted in accordance with ARI-575-95 are the *averaged* A-weighted sound level in dBA and the *averaged* octave-band sound pressure levels 1 m from the equipment surfaces. The point-to-point data should also be available upon request.

Equipment Operating Points for Sound Rating

ARI Standard 575-95 recommends that water-cooled chillers be rated at full load or at a mutually agreed upon load point. Because chiller noise can vary considerably over a map of typical operating points, most manufacturers can provide data, if requested, over a range of condensing temperatures, pressures, and capacities.

Frequency Range of Available Data

Octave mid-band frequencies from 63 Hz to 8000 Hz.

Most Important Octave Bands in Product Application

Bands containing tonal components, as shown in Table 15-2.

Differences in Acoustical Quality of Chillers

The sound quality attributes of the four types of chillers discussed above are distinctly different. The quietest and least subjectively annoying chiller is the absorption machine because of the absence of prominent tonal components in the typical sound spectrum. Screw chillers tend to be the most annoying due to strong tonal content.

Variability of Data

As with any laboratory test procedure, there are always measurement uncertainties to be taken into account when reporting data. Experience indicates that uncertainties in the probable accuracy of measurements, as shown in Table 15-3, should be considered when applying manufacturers' test data to an HVAC system design.

TABLE 15-3
Estimated Variability of Product Sound Pressure Data Due to Measurement Uncertainties and Production Quality Control
The Frequency Bands Most Affected by Chiller Load are Indicated by Shading[a]

Water Cooled Chillers						
Octave Mid-Band Frequency Hz	Measurement Uncertainty of ARI 575 Test Procedure[b] dB	Repeatability of Test Data[c] dB	Production Variability[d] dB	Cumulative Uncertainty Due To All Previous Factors[e] dB	Variability of Random Sample *re* Catalog in Free Field[f] dB	Bands Most Affected by Chiller Load dB
63	± 3	± 2	± 4	± 4	+6, –0	
125	± 3	± 1	± 3	± 3	+5, –0	
250-500	± 2	± 1	± 3	± 4	+3, –0	
1000-4000	± 1.5	± 1	± 3	± 4	+3, –0	see Table 15-6
8000	± 2.5	± 0.5	± 3	± 5	+3, –0	see Table 15-6

a. The size and amount of absorption in the mechanical equipment room affects the measured sound pressure level, as indicated in Table 15-5.
b. Estimated standard deviation includes variations due to different operators, measurement location, and instrumentation. (Based on data in ANSI Standard S12.10)
c. Repetitive testing of same unit in same laboratory.
d. Subject to manufacturing tolerances permitted in production quality control.
e. Based on the square root of the sum of the squares of all uncertainties.
f. Published catalog data are not customarily derived from a statistical sampling of production units but usually are determined by testing a prototype. Thus, the results of testing random production samples would tend to exceed those published by the manufacturer.

Variability of point-to-point data in ARI-575 tests

As pointed out earlier, published ARI 575-95 sound data are derived by averaging measurements at a number of specified test points around the chiller. Typically, for most water chillers, the point-to-point variation in A-weighted sound level (dBA) is about ±3 dB to 5 dB with respect to the space-averaged value. The maximum levels encountered are often located closest to the compressor discharge line; the minimum levels usually occur at the ends of the condenser and evaporator shells.

This variability should be recognized when making measurements qualifying a field installation because it might not be feasible to duplicate the exact test points specified by ARI 575-95. When making field measurements to verify manufacturers' data, if the equipment room is large enough (see Table 15-3) and the equipment is located such that it is possible to duplicate the specified measurement points, the energy-averaged octave-band data should be in nominal agreement with those published by the manufacturer. However, in small to medium-sized mechanical rooms, good agreement is unlikely because the reverberant buildup can be substantial.

Furthermore, if tonal components are present (typical of all chiller types except the absorption machine), there may be significant differences between the data measured at a single point, such as opposite the compressor discharge line, and the energy-average of all points around the equipment. In the worst case, "standing-wave" patterns caused by strong interference effects due to wall reflections may produce changes in sound pressure level on the order of 10 dB to 15 dB with incremental changes in the microphone position of only 1 ft.

Under no circumstances should one expect to validate a manufacturer's data by making a single measurement at a worst-case point; the manufacturers' data typically represent the log-average of some 20 measurement points for a reasonably sized chiller. As one example, a comparison on a screw chiller between manufacturers' data and a single worst-case measurement in a large mechanical room is shown in Table 15-4. It should be noted that due to the small reverberant buildup close to the machine in a large mechanical room, reasonable agreement can be expected in the octave bands above 250 Hz. However, in the case of a screw compressor, the pure-tone lobe-passage frequency typically occurs in the 250 Hz octave-band and the single-point level at one location may be 14 dB greater than the space-average level.

TABLE 15-4
Comparison of Manufacturers' Free-Field Data with ARI 575-95 Data at a Single Location for a Screw Chiller

Octave-Band Sound Pressure Level of Screw Chiller							
Octave Band	63	125	250	500	1k	2k	4k
Energy-Averaged ARI 575 Data @ 1m	80	80	92	92	90	84	77
Single-Point @ 1 m from Compressor	76	85	106	90	91	84	79
Difference	–4 dB	+5 dB	+14 dB	–2 dB	+1 dB	+ 0 dB	+2 dB

APPLICATION OF WATER CHILLER SOUND DATA TO HVAC SYSTEMS

KNOW THE CONDITIONS UNDER WHICH THE SUBMITTED CHILLER SOUND DATA WERE OBTAINED

A majority of the equipment sound rating data discussed in this book are expressed in terms of sound power level, which is essentially independent of the acoustical environment in which the product is tested or will be installed in an application. However, ARI Standard 575-95 sound data are expressed in terms of sound pressure level, averaged over a number of measurement points. Since sound pressure level data are dependent upon the acoustical environment in which the measurements are made, increases on the order of 10 dB to 15 dB can occur when comparing data for the same chiller rated by the manufacturer in a quasi-outdoor environment with those obtained from measurements in a smaller mechanical room in the field.

Figure 15-3 illustrates a problem that exists when using typical manufacturers' sound data based on ARI Standard 575 to predict the sound level of the equipment when installed in a typical mechanical equipment room. Manufacturers' sound level data are often measured in a large test room or in an outdoor location where the effects of wall reflections are minimized, as in Figure 15-3a, whereas the room in a typical field installation is usually both hard and highly reflective, as illustrated in Figure 15-3b. This level of confusion occurs because the ARI Standard 575-95 specifies only the method of measurement but not the acoustical environment in which tests are to be conducted.

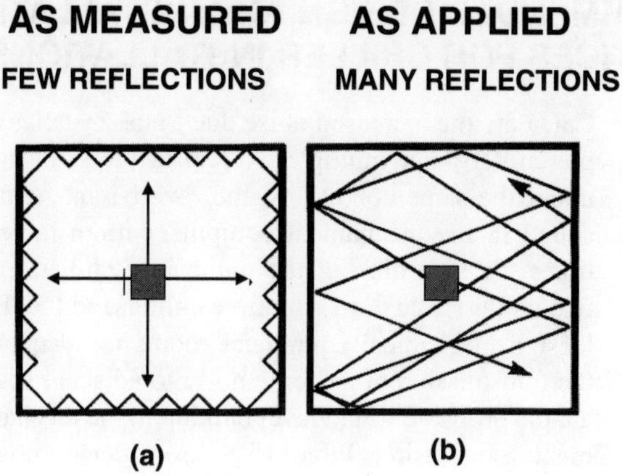

FIGURE 15-3 Sound propagation pattern in free-field room with no reflections compared to that in a typical mechanical room with reflective walls and ceiling.

Table 15-5 shows the anticipated sound buildup in hard mechanical equipment rooms that have little acoustical absorption as compared with mechanical equipment rooms with sound absorption added on the perimeter walls (ISO 1981). In this example, it is assumed that at least 2 in. thick absorptive sidewall treatment is to be used on the mechanical equipment room walls when either reciprocating or screw chillers are installed, whereas 1 in. absorptive sidewall treatment is usually sufficient for the installation of centrifugal chillers.

TABLE 15-5

Typical Buildup[a] of A-Weighted Sound Level (dBA) with Chillers Installed in (MER) Mechanical Equipment Rooms of Various Sizes

Chiller Location	Typical Volume of Chiller Space ft^3	With Sidewall Absorption Add	With No Sidewall Absorption Add
Outdoors	∞	N/A	+ 0 dB
Large Factory Space	100000	N/A	+ 0 dB
Large MER	50000	+ 0 dB	+ 2 dB
Medium MER	25000	+ 2-4 dB	+ 8-10 dB
Small MER	5000	+ 7-11 dB	+ 13-15 dB

a. Table based on equation:

$$\text{dB buildup} = 10 \cdot \log\{1 + 4 \cdot (\text{measurement box area/MER surface area}) \cdot (1 - \alpha)/\alpha\}$$

where α is the average sabine absorption coefficient of the mechanical equipment room (MER).

RECOMMENDED DESIGN AND INSTALLATION PRACTICES FOR CHILLER INSTALLATIONS

- Calculate the increased noise due to the installation of multiple chillers. For multiple chillers of the same type running under the same conditions, the reverberant field buildup of sound in the mechanical equipment room increases as ten times the logarithm of the number of chillers running. For two chillers, add 3 dB; for three chillers, add 5 dB; etc.
- Design mechanical equipment rooms to adequately control the transmission of airborne noise to adjacent spaces. Evaluate the probable sound level buildup in the mechanical equipment room using Table 15-5. Consider adding acoustical absorption to the walls and/or ceiling of the mechanical equipment room to reduce sound level buildup.
- Seek application assistance from the manufacturer for noise control options such as optional internal silencers or external lagging of the compressor discharge line and condenser shells. Figure 15-4 illustrates that not all parts of a centrifugal chiller package radiate the same sound power. The discharge line and condenser shell are often the dominant noise radiators.
- Be aware that large differences in acoustical quality exist among various types of chillers.
- Chiller loading affects sound level. Evaluate manufacturers' data at multiple load points to determine whether the noise criterion assigned an adjacent occupied space can be met over the anticipated load range of operation.

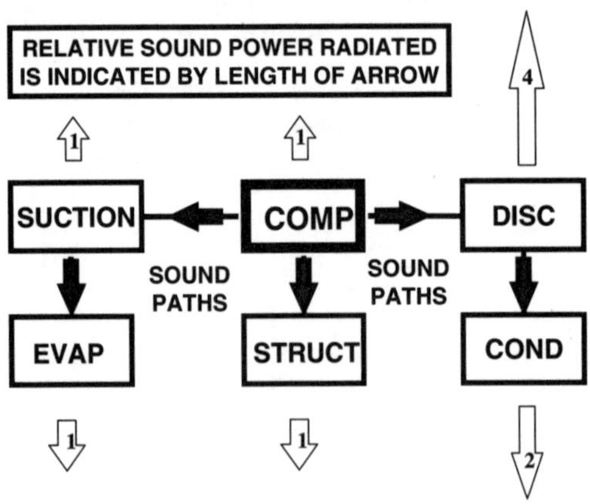

FIGURE 15-4 Relative sound power radiated by a centrifugal chiller.

TABLE 15-6
Chiller Vibration Isolation Recommendations

Chiller Type	On or Below Grade	Above Grade
Absorption	Not required	Ribbed neoprene pad[a]
Reciprocating	1 in. static deflection springs over ribbed neoprene pad[b]	Springs over double layers of ribbed neoprene pad[c,d]
Screw	1 in. static deflection springs over ribbed neoprene pad[e]	Same as above
Centrifugal	Ribbed neoprene pad[d]	Same as above

a. Single-thickness pad. Recommended loading to 40-50 psi.
b. Laterally stable spring isolator with ribbed neoprene base pad loaded 40-50 psi.
c. Spring static deflection should be at least 8 times incremental floor static deflection due to added weight of chiller.
d. Inertia bases may also be considered in critical applications.
e. All ribbed neoprene pads to be ribbed on both surfaces. Neoprene pads waffled on both sides may also be used.

VIBRATION ISOLATION CONSIDERATIONS

Neoprene flexible connectors are recommended at connections to condenser water and chilled water supply and return piping as one method to control structureborne noise transmission via the piping. Flexible conduit is also recommended for connecting all electrical and control wiring, and flexible connectors are required by building codes for vent piping. Short circuiting of equipment vibration isolators by nonisolated floor supports of connected water piping is a common installation oversight and must be avoided.

Table 15-6 lists the typical vibration isolation recommendations[3] for water chiller equipment. The reader is referred to Chapter 43 of the *1995 ASHRAE Handbook—Applications* for more detailed recommendations, particularly for installations in long-span structural systems.

3. All ribbed neoprene pads to be ribbed on both surfaces. Neoprene pads waffled on both sides may also be used.

SUGGESTED NOISE AND VIBRATION ISOLATION SPECIFICATIONS

Noise Specifications

Noise specifications for chillers typically have two purposes:

1. OSHA
2. Noise criteria

OSHA

To address OSHA[4] noise exposure concerns for persons working in the mechanical equipment room. For this case, a simple not-to-exceed maximum A-weighted sound level (dBA) specified for all load conditions is sufficient. The following specification is suggested:

All chillers scheduled below shall have been tested in the manufacturer's facility in complete accordance with the latest revision of ARI Standard 575, Method of Measuring Machinery Sound Within an Equipment Space. *The Average A-weighted sound pressure levels, defined in the standard, shall not exceed the sound pressure levels scheduled below at any load capacity between 25% and 100% of design.*

When Tested in Accordance with ARI Standard 575, the Averaged A-Weighted Sound Level Shall Not Exceed the Following Values When Tested in the Manufacturer's Facility[a]	
MARK	**Average A- Weighted Sound Level (dBA) @ 1 meter**
CH-1	xx dBA
CH-2	xx dBA

a. See Table 15-3 for dBA increases to be expected in mechanical equipment rooms.

Part Load Conditions

Some chillers produce more noise at partial load than at full load. Therefore, specify the maximum sound pressure levels at all operating conditions. Table 15-7 shows expected level variation over the typical load range of the various chiller types.

---

4. If the time-weighted average noise exposure is greater than 85 dBA, OSHA regulations require the initiation of a hearing conservation program. If the time-weighted average exposure is greater than 90 dBA, the use of engineering noise controls are mandated.

TABLE 15-7
Chiller Noise Characteristics

Chiller Type	Where Min. Noise Occurs	Where Max. Noise Occurs	Typical Difference (Max. To Min.)
Reciprocating	Full load	With compressors unloaded	2-3 dBA
Centrifugal	Full load	Part load	5 dBA
Screw	Design conditions	Part load conditions furthest from design conditions	6 dBA

To Meet Noise Criteria

To specify the maximum octave-band noise levels in the mechanical room consistent with an assigned noise criterion, the following specification is suggested:

All chillers scheduled below shall have been tested in complete accordance with the latest revision of ARI Standard 575, Method of Measuring Machinery Sound Within an Equipment Space. *The representative octave-band sound pressure levels, defined in the standard, shall not exceed the sound pressure levels scheduled below at any load capacity between 25% and 100% of design.*

When Tested in Accordance with ARI Standard 575, the Averaged Octave-Band Sound Pressure Levels (dB) @ 1 Meter Octave Mid-Band Frequency in Hz							
Mark	**63**	**125**	**250**	**500**	**1k**	**2k**	**4k**
CH-1							
CH-2							

VIBRATION ISOLATION SPECIFICATIONS

Vibration isolation should be in accordance with Table 42, Chapter 43, *1995 ASHRAE Handbook—Applications.*

REFERENCES

ISO. 1981. *ISO Standard 3744, Acoustics—Determination of sound power levels of noise sources*. Annex A, "Engineering methods for free field conditions over a reflecting plane." Geneva: International Organization for Standardization.

Chapter 16
Cooling Towers

by *Charles Ebbing and Warren Blazier*

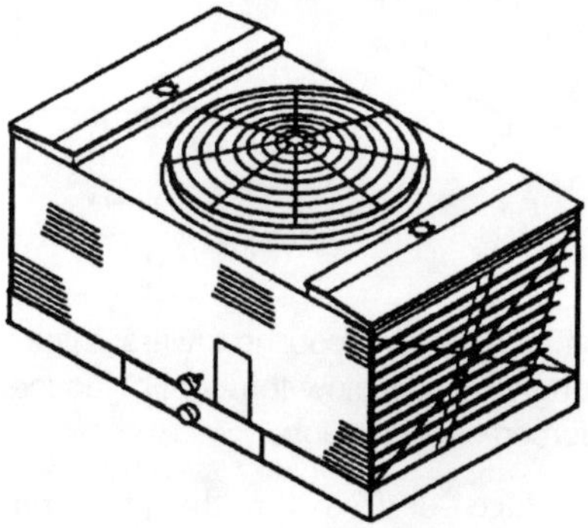

OVERVIEW

Common Cooling Tower Types and Their Noise Characteristics

The most common type of cooling tower is the induced-draft, or draw-through, tower. This type of tower consists of a propeller fan at the top of the tower for the induction of air, a water distribution system and a cooling system, a water collecting basin, and air intake louvers on one to four sides of the tower structure. The propeller fan and its drive motor with speed reduction mechanism (gear or belts) are usually mounted on a unitized frame.

A forced-draft, or blow-through, tower differs from the induced-draft tower because air is forced through the tower media by the use of either centrifugal or axial fans side-mounted on the tower or with a propeller fan beneath a somewhat raised tower. These types of towers are shown in Figure 16-1.

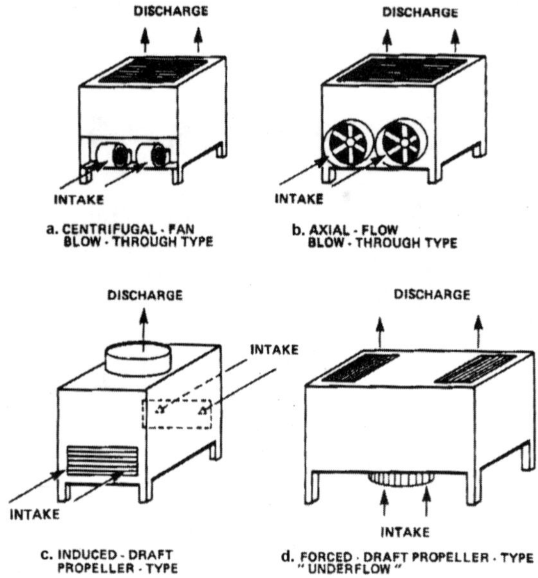

FIGURE 16-1 Common types of cooling towers: a) centrifugal blow-through, b) axial blow-through, c) induced draw-through, d) forced blow-through.

With an induced-draft tower, the predominant noise at the tower discharge is produced by the fan. This fan noise is emitted in both an upward direction and along the ground-plane, normal to the air intake louvers. In addition, water splashing noise is emitted from the intake louvers. When the fan is off, waterfall noise increases and is apparent at much greater distances than with the fan on since the water is free fall, not opposed by airflow.

Usually the noise of a propeller-type tower includes a low frequency blade-passage tone in the range of the 31.5 Hz or 63 Hz octave mid-band frequency, in addition to broad-band noise extending over the remainder of the spectrum with a slope that decreases at a rate of 3 to 4 dB/octave. The waterfall noise is also broad band in character, but it is usually only noticeable in all frequency ranges above 125 Hz.

With a propeller fan serving a forced-draft tower, the primary difference relative to an induced-draft application is that the noise at the air intake is principally fan noise, and the air intake area extends around the lower perimeter of the tower near the ground or roof-plane on which the tower is situated. The fan noise is radiated equally in all four directions along the ground or roof-plane, and from the tower discharge, slightly reduced as a result of losses in passing through the tower media.

With both of these tower types, the fan noise level for a given model increases approximately in direct proportion to the fan horsepower. However, the fan noise of any model is strongly dependent upon the propeller tip speed. Although tip speeds in the past have typically been in the range of 51 m/s to 61 m/s (10,000 ft/min to 12,000 ft/min), for noise control reasons propeller tip speeds are often reduced in design stages by 10% to 40%. However, the lower operating noise level may be partially offset if tower size has to be increased to meet the required cooling capacity. Also, the water splash noise for any one tower model increases directly with water flow rate.

Reducing Tower Noise

- The strategy employed to reduce fan noise is to first replace the standard fan with one having a higher fan tip solidity, usually with more blades. At the airflow required to deliver the rated capacity of the tower, the new fan will operate at lower speed and at approximately the same horsepower, but it will generate less noise. Of course, it is usually more costly.
- The second most cost effective step in the sound reduction strategy is to add attenuation to the air intake and/or discharge.
- The third most cost effective step is to oversize the tower so the larger than necessary fan can be operated slower.

When centrifugal or axial fans are used in a forced-draft tower, the inlet fan noise is radiated directly from the air intakes parallel to the ground-plane. However, the fan discharge noise, which is only slightly attenuated by passage through the tower media, combines with waterfall noise and radiates vertically from the top of the tower. The fan noise in towers of this type is fairly broad band, but blade-passage tonal components may also be present. Axial fans on a forced-draft tower produce maximum sound levels in the frequency range (250 Hz to 1000 Hz octave bands). Centrifugal fans usually produce maximum levels in the 125 Hz to 500 Hz octave bands for air foil or backwardly inclined blades and 1000 Hz to 2000 Hz octave bands for forward-curved blades.

Generally, for these types of towers, waterfall noise will not be significant except for observers located directly above or adjacent to the tower.

TABLE 16-1

Directional Factors for Cooling Tower Noise[a]

Oct. Band (Hz)	31.5	63	125	250	500	1000	2000	4000	8000
Centrifugal Fan Blow-Through Tower									
Front (Fan inlet)	+3	+3	+2	+3	+4	+3	+2	+2	+2
Side (Enclosed)	+0	+0	+0	–2	–3	–4	–5	–5	–5
Rear (Enclosed)	+0	+0	–1	–2	–3	–4	–5	–6	–6
Top (Discharge)	–3	–3	–2	+0	+1	+2	+3	+4	+5
Axial Blow-Through Tower									
Front (Fan Inlet)	+2	+2	+4	+6	+6	+5	+5	+5	+5
Side (Enclosed)	+1	+1	+1	–2	–5	–5	–5	–5	–4
Rear (Enclosed)	–3	–3	–4	–7	–7	–7	–8	–11	–8
Top (Discharge)	–5	–5	–5	–5	–2	+0	+0	+2	+1
Induced-Draft Propeller-Type Tower									
Front (Air Inlet)	+0	+0	+0	+1	+2	+2	+2	+3	+3
Side (Enclosed)	–3	–3	–3	–3	–3	–3	–4	–5	–6
Top (Discharge)	+3	+3	+3	+3	+3	+4	+4	+3	+3
"Underflow" Forced-Draft Propeller-Type Tower									
Any Side	–1	–1	–1	–2	–2	–3	–3	–4	–4
Top	+2	+2	+2	+3	+3	+4	+4	+5	+5

a. Air intakes for induced-draft towers may be located on one to all four sides. In the latter case, the L_p in each of four directions would be the average L_p as there would be no directional factor for the air intake.

NOISE CHARACTERISTICS OF COOLING TOWERS

DIRECTIVITY OF COOLING TOWER NOISE EMISSION

To estimate the octave-band sound pressure level, L_p, at a particular distance and direction from a cooling tower based on published sound power level, L_w, two steps are required. First, it is necessary to calculate the average L_p in each octave by subtracting the attenuation factor due to hemispherical spreading and atmospheric absorption for the distance from source to receiver. Second, because cooling towers do not radiate noise uniformly in all directions, as illustrated in Figure 16-2, it is necessary to add the corrections given in Table 16-1 to the calculated average L_p. However, these corrections should not be added at close-in positions, such as less than 10 ft, or where there are nearby reflecting or obstructing surfaces that might modify the normal radiation pattern of tower noise.

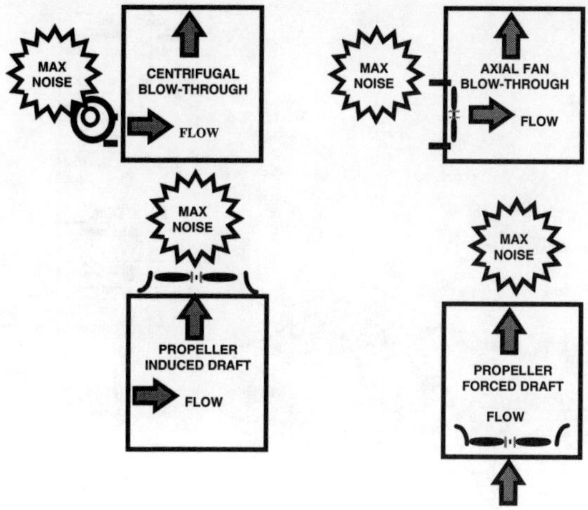

FIGURE 16-2 Direction of maximum noise radiation for various types of cooling towers.

MANUFACTURERS' SOUND RATING PROCEDURES AND PRACTICES FOR COOLING TOWERS

The Cooling Tower Institute Code ATC-128 (CTI 1981) is the primary test method used to measure the cooling tower noise. In this procedure, the tower is located in a free field above a reflecting surface and operated at design conditions and at design fan power and speed. If these design conditions cannot be met, then agreed-upon conditions must be reported. The test does not dictate how the operating point is controlled. The test specifies measurements of sound pressure levels, L_p, in octave bands at distances equal to or greater than 50 ft from the air-inlet face and at 5 ft above the ground. The octave-band levels from 63 Hz to 8k Hz are measured around the tower at uniform intervals. These data are corrected for any influence by background noise. There must be no reflecting surfaces near the measurement microphone.[1] At least two manufacturers measure at other than the suggested distances. A typical set of data supplied by a cooling tower manufacturer is shown in Figure 16-3.

1. If the measurement for the prototype is measured in a free field and then installed near reflecting surfaces, increased noise levels can result. Furthermore, the directivity higher than 5 ft above grade is not accounted for.

Top SPL (dB)

Octave Band	Distance 5 Ft.	Distance 50 Ft.
1	100	79
2	97	80
3	94	79
4	88	77
5	80	70
6	73	65
7	69	62
8	62	59
dB(A)	90	77

Air Inlet SPL (dB)

Octave Band	Distance 5 Ft.	Distance 50 Ft.
1	86	71
2	87	73
3	85	71
4	84	71
5	80	67
6	70	61
7	61	56
8	55	50
dB(A)	85	72

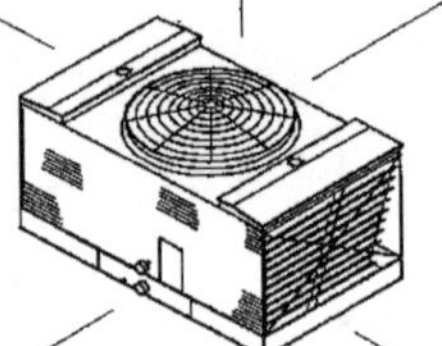

End SPL (dB)

Octave Band	Distance 5 Ft.	Distance 50 Ft.
1	81	74
2	84	73
3	82	71
4	78	70
5	71	64
6	63	55
7	61	53
8	58	45
dB(A)	78	70

End SPL (dB)

Octave Band	Distance 5 Ft.	Distance 50 Ft.
1	81	74
2	84	73
3	82	71
4	78	70
5	71	64
6	63	55
7	61	53
8	58	45
dB(A)	78	70

Air Inlet SPL (dB)

Octave Band	Distance 5 Ft.	Distance 50 Ft.
1	86	71
2	87	73
3	85	71
4	84	71
5	80	67
6	70	61
7	61	56
8	55	50
dB(A)	85	72

Calculated PWL

Octave Band	(dB)
1	107
2	105
3	103
4	102
5	98
6	93
7	86
8	84

FIGURE 16-3 Typical sound data provided by one manufacturer.

TEST FACILITIES USED TO OBTAIN DATA

Sound pressure measurements are typically made outdoors in a free field above a reflecting plane.

CALCULATED SOUND DATA

Octave-band and A-weighted sound power levels are calculated from 50 ft sound pressure data.

DATA RATING POINTS

Typical data supplied are with the fan operating at full speed and with the fan operating at half speed (for two-speed motors). The number of blades for the propeller fans and their operating speed are necessary to determine blade-passing frequency, but most manufacturers do not publish these.

FREQUENCY RANGE OF DATA

- 63 Hz to 8000 Hz octave bands.

Most Important Bands in Product Application

- Meeting maximum noise limits 63 Hz to 2000 Hz.
- Obtaining best acoustical quality 31.5 Hz to 250 Hz.

Ratings in Terms of Sound Pressure

Measured sound pressure level data are provided by most manufacturers at distances of 5 ft and 50 ft from all sides and the top of the tower.

Ratings in Terms of Sound Power (L_W)

Octave-band sound power level data are derived from the measured 50 ft octave-band sound pressure levels by summing the data on an energy basis at each 50 ft location and adding 25 dB[2] to the summed level in each octave band.

Data Quality

Not all manufacturers' data are of equal quality, and the user is cautioned to determine the basis upon which the supplied data was obtained before using them to predict the result for a specific installation. Data supplied by manufacturers may be derived by any one or combination of the following procedures:

- Data measured on a test unit of the specified model.
- Data obtained on some or all models regressed into a set of equations that allows sound data to be reliably estimated for any model.
- Data that are based on cooling tower units that have had recent design modifications that may or may not significantly change the noise ratings.

Users should question any data that are not traceable to one of the above procedures.

Manufacturers' data are often available in one-third octave bands, although only octave-band sound power data at 63 Hz and above is presently published by the industry. If one-third octave-band data are required to determine the presence of significant tonal components, they can often be obtained from many of the tower manufacturers.

---

2. This derives from $r = 50$ ft or 15.2 m. Then $10 \times \log(2\pi r^2) = 20 \times \log(15.2) + 10 \times \log(2\pi) = 31.6$. Furthermore, the average pressure = log summation of five pressures minus $10 \times \log(5) = 7$. Hence, $31.6 - 7 = 24.6$ dB.

Uncertainties in the Application of Manufacturers' Data

There are several factors that can affect the reliability of manufacturers' data. Table 16-2 lists uncertainties that should be recognized in field application of the data. Sound pressure levels measured at the job site usually correlate well with the manufacturer's data if job site conditions are similar to those under which the unit was tested.

APPLICATION OF COOLING TOWER SOUND RATINGS

Effect of Distances Greater Than 50 ft

To estimate the sound pressure levels at distances greater than 50 ft, the attenuation of sound pressure levels for distances greater than 50 ft is shown in Table 16-3. Table 16-3 includes the effect of high-frequency absorption by the air for distances greater than 100 ft. For distances greater than about 500 ft, wind and temperature gradients in the air also have an effect, but the effects are too complicated

Table 16-2
Estimates of the Variability of Sound Pressure Data

Cooling Towers					
Octave Mid-Band Frequency	**Expected Repeatability of Units Tested in Outdoors**[a]	**Expected Range Between Different Samples of "Identical Product"**[b]	**Expected Range Due To All Previous Factors**[c]	**Expected Difference Between a Typical Sample and Catalog Data**	**Bands Most Affected by Nearby Reflective Surfaces**
63	±2 dB	±3 dB	±4 dB	+6, -0	see Table 16-5
125	±2 dB	±3 dB	±4 dB	+5, -0	
250	±2 dB	±3 dB	±4 dB	+3, -0	
500-4000	±2 dB	±3 dB	±4 dB	+3, -0	
8000	±2 dB	±3 dB	±4dB	+3, -0	

a. Estimated standard deviation includes variations due to different operators, measurement location, and instrumentation (based on data in ANSI Std. S12.10).
b. Repetitive testing of same unit in same testing location.
c. Based on square root of the sum of the squares of uncertainties.

TABLE 16-3
Attenuation for Distances Greater than 50 ft
Subtract These Values for the 50 ft Data to Estimate Levels at Other Distances from Tower Face.

Distance (ft)	63	125	250	500	1000	2000	4000	8000
50	0	0	0	0	0	0	0	0
63	2	2	2	2	2	2	2	2
80	4	4	4	4	4	4	4	4
100	6	6	6	6	6	6	6	6
125	8	8	8	8	8	8	9	10
160	10	10	10	10	10	10	11	12
200	12	12	12	12	12	13	14	15
250	14	14	14	14	14	15	16	18
320	16	16	16	16	16	17	18	21
400	18	18	18	18	19	19	21	24
500	20	20	20	20	21	22	24	27
630	22	22	22	22	23	24	27	31
800	24	24	24	25	25	26	30	35
1000	26	26	26	27	27	29	34	40
1250	28	28	28	29	30	32	38	46
1600	30	30	30	31	32	35	43	53
2000	32	32	32	33	35	38	47	61
2500	34	34	34	36	38	42	53	70

and the occurrences too variable to consider here. Use this table to estimate the attenuation under calm weather conditions without significant thermal gradients encountered on clear sunny days.

ESTIMATING SOUND LEVELS BETWEEN 50 FT AND 5 FT

To estimate the sound pressure levels between 50 ft and 5 ft, Table 16-4 can be used to determine corrections to be applied to the 50 ft data.

BUILD-UP OF CLOSE-IN NOISE LEVELS

When cooling towers are located close to a wall or inside a space formed by two or three surrounding walls, the principal concern may be with noise in the immediate vicinity (within 5 ft to 10 ft)

TABLE 16-4
Estimating Noise Levels at Distances Between 5 ft and 50 ft Using 50 ft Data (Adapted from BAC 1971)

Distance from Tower Face	dB to Add to 50 ft Sound Levels
50	0
45	1
40	1
35	2
30	3
25	4
20	5
15	7
10	9
5	12

TABLE 16-5
Effect of Nearby Reflective Surfaces on 5 ft Cooling Tower Noise Levels

Nearby Reflecting Surfaces Present	dB Adder to 5 ft Data for Nearby Reflections
None	0 dB
Single Building Wall within 10 ft of Tower	3 dB
Open Courtyard	5 dB
Mechanical Equipment Room	5 dB - 15 dB

of the cooling tower rather than the reflected noise radiated to some more remote location. If the area of the reflecting surfaces near the tower is at least three times the area of the closest tower surface and is closer than half the distance from the closest tower face to the point of concern, then the actual noise level can be greater than expected (Miller 1991). Table 16-5 shows the estimated effects of nearby reflective surfaces on the 5 ft cooling tower noise levels.

RECOMMENDED DESIGN AND INSTALLATION PRACTICES FOR COOLING TOWERS

COOLING TOWER LOCATION GUIDANCE

Cooling towers are often situated near the perimeter of a site and near the property line, adjacent to a building, or on a rooftop, depending on the cooling tower size. The choice of tower location is an important first step in the noise control design process. The location should be as far as possible from sound sensitive receivers, and, if possible, the top discharge area of the tower should not be directly visible by a receiver.

An important early item in determining the acceptability of cooling tower noise in a given environment is to select a noise control goal, or criterion, appropriate to the land-use of concern. If a local noise ordinance mandates maximum octave-band sound pressure levels or maximum A-weighted sound levels, this may be the goal to consider. However, if the intrusion of cooling tower noise is significantly above that of the normal background or ambient noise level due to other sources in the area, a situation that is unacceptable to persons living nearby may develop. In many instances, the avoidance of noise complaints often requires that the level of the intruding noise be much lower than that specified by a local ordinance. Because the cost of correcting a tower noise problem after the fact can approach or exceed the original cost of the installation, it is always advisable to consider the noise level impact in the early stages of planning and prior to making a tower selection.

When locating cooling towers on the top of a building, it is advisable to position the tower over the least acoustically sensitive areas, such as unoccupied spaces. The need to vibration isolate the tower and connected piping requires evaluation early in the design process because the noise criterion for the spaces directly below may not be achievable unless the system is vibration isolated. Furthermore, the noise of a rooftop installation may propagate to other nearby commercial or residential buildings at or above the elevation of the tower. In such instances, the addition of sound attenuators on the intake and discharge sides of the tower, or the installation of barriers in the source-to-receiver path, may be required.

Cooling Tower Noise Control by Tower Design

Avoiding Tower Start-Up Noises

Belt squeal

Belt squeal and the banging noises produced by the sudden starting torque applied to the fan-drive system can create noise complaints about tower operation. Belt squeal at start-up normally implies improper belt tension or adjustment and usually can be controlled by proper maintenance practices.

Soft starters

If normal maintenance does not correct the problem, the installation of "soft-start" capacitor-run motors or a variable frequency drive may be required. Today soft-start starters for conventional induction motors are available from most starter manufacturers, and they are much smaller and more cost effective than special motors or variable speed drives. These are commonly used to solve complaints having to do with airborne and structureborne start-up noises.

Fan Speed Control Considerations

Single-speed tower

Single-speed cooling towers are least obtrusive if running continuously. It is frequently the cyclic nature of an operation that triggers a noise complaint.

Two-speed towers

The most frequent complaints about cooling tower noise are likely to occur at night when the ambient noise is lower than during the daytime hours. Because the cooling load requirements for the tower are significantly reduced at night in many applications, operating the cooling tower fans at part-speed during these periods can result in a sizable noise reduction. Since fan noise is approximately proportional to the fifth power of the tip speed, two-speed fan motors are often installed to correct nighttime complaints.

Reducing the fan speed as capacity is reduced can also reduce the frequency of tower start-up noises, which are a potential source of complaints. Propeller fan towers operating at half speed can result in A-weighted sound level reductions of as much as 8 dBA to 10 dBA (BAC 1971). For example, in a two-tower installation, it is significantly quieter to run two towers at half speed during the reduced nighttime capacity requirement than it is to operate only one at full speed. Because of the substantial reduction in fan noise that occurs as speed is lowered, two cooling towers operating at one-half fan speed produce about 8 dBA less noise than one tower alone operating at full speed.

Use of variable frequency drive (VFD)

Add-on packages for cooling tower noise control include the use of variable frequency drives. This may improve overall energy efficiency, minimize start-up noise, allow speed reduction at night to reduce nighttime noise, and allow gradual speed changes with demand capacity to minimize the noticeability of sudden speed changes.

Capacity control options: Oversizing of the tower

In some applications, and particularly HVAC systems, the full tower capacity will not be required during the more acoustically critical nighttime hours. In such cases, it may be feasible to operate the tower fan at half speed or use a VFD to provide quieter operation during these off-peak hours. However, if the conditions are such that full capacity must be maintained at all hours, a special, more costly fan may be selected for propeller fan units to operate at a lower speed and thereby reduce the tower noise level by 3 dBA to 5 dBA. If greater reduction in noise is required, the tower (propeller or centrifugal fan) can be oversized to operate at significantly reduced fan speed for noise reductions of up to 12 dBA. Both special fans and oversized towers can be employed with speed control to effect further noise reductions during acoustically sensitive periods.

Path Noise Control (Outdoors)

For Noise-Sensitive Rooftop Applications

For cooling towers located on rooftops, try to locate units over nonsensitive spaces.

Addition of Sound Attenuators on Intake and Discharge of Tower

Conventional duct type sound attenuators can present a substantial additional pressure drop to the fan if not carefully selected. Overcoming the sound attenuator pressure drop may require that the fan be operated at a higher speed to achieve the rated cooling capacity of the tower. This, in turn, adds to the sound emission from the fan and destroys a major portion of the attenuation effect. Some cooling tower manufacturers have developed special purpose sound attenuators and deflectors for their equipment that add very little to the fan static pressure requirement. However, because of the size and expense, the designer should first attempt to achieve an installation that will be satisfactory from a sound standpoint without the need to apply external silencers.

Using Barriers (Free Standing, Buildings, or Natural Barrier)

Specially constructed barriers can be used to control cooling tower noise. Also, buildings or parts of buildings, and earth berms or other formations, can also be used to as attenuation devices.

TABLE 16-6
Approximate Insertion Loss of Cooling Tower Barriers

Octave Band Insertion Loss of Barrier (dB)									
Barrier Type	**31.5**	**63**	**125**	**250**	**500**	**1000**	**2000**	**4000**	**8000**
Barrier that Blocks Line of Sight	5	5	5	5	5	6	7	8	9
Barrier that Extends 3 ft to 5 ft in All Directions	5	5	5	6	7	9	11	13	16

Table 16-6 shows a simplified barrier attenuation (BAC 1971). It presents the insertion loss of a solid barrier without air leaks with a surface density of more than 4 lb/ft^2, constructed close to the tower that just shields the tower from view and breaks the line of sight. Also included is the insertion loss of a barrier that extends 3 ft to 5 ft beyond the line of sight.

VIBRATION ISOLATION CONSIDERATIONS

Locate the unit over the most rigid part of the structural building supports, as illustrated in Figure 16-4. Adequate structural rigidity can be best obtained by extending pipe columns from building columns and placing steel members on top of the pipe columns. Avoid locating cooling towers on roof curbs in the center of column bays.

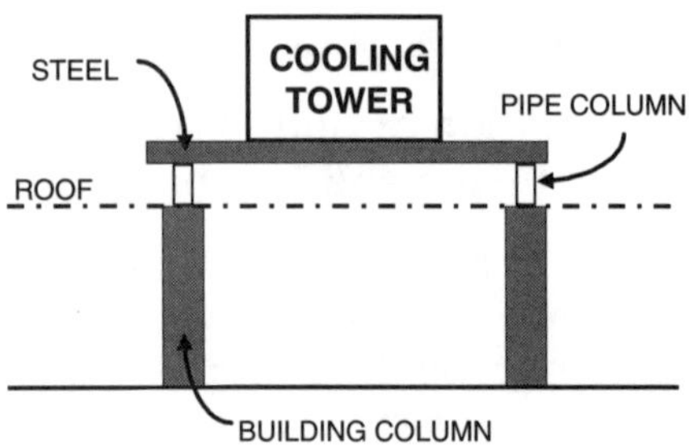

FIGURE 16-4 Best structural support for cooling towers.

When a tower is mounted on a building, the designer must ensure that adequate vibration isolation is provided. To do this, the incremental deflection of the roof (how much the roof deflects with the tower installed) must be less than one-eighth the static deflection of the vibration isolator (Mason 1966). For example, if the incremental deflection of the roof is 0.2 in., then the static deflection of the isolator must be at least 1.6 in. In some cases where the tower is installed on roof spans greater than 30 ft, isolators with static deflection less than 2 in. will be inadequate. The designer needs to follow ASHRAE guidelines (1995) for vibration isolation of cooling towers and tower water lines.

If the tower is to be operated over a noise-sensitive space, consider the use of a concrete pad, equivalent to 6 in. thick dense concrete, under the tower extended out to at least 3 ft beyond the tower footprint.

If a VFD system is used to operate the fans, it is important to lock out the control system to prevent the fan speed from operating near the resonant frequency of the vibration isolation system supporting the tower. In a theoretical sense, the ratio of minimum fan speed, rps (rpm/60), to the isolator natural frequency, Hz, should be about 1.4 to avoid the magnification of cooling tower vibration on its mounting system. However, in practice ratios of 1.2 do not seem to create significant problems. Since typical cooling tower mounting systems have natural frequencies in the range of 2 Hz to 4 Hz, designing to a ratio of 1.4 limits the fan speed to about 170 rpm for the 2 Hz isolation system and 340 rpm for the 4 Hz isolation system. The minimum fan speeds using a ratio of 1.2 would be about 145 rpm and 290 rpm for the 2 Hz and 4 Hz isolation systems, respectively. Thus, if a VFD drive is used, the natural frequency of the vibration isolation system must be chosen to avoid interference at the lowest contemplated fan speed.

TRANSMISSION LOSS CONSIDERATIONS

When a cooling tower is roof mounted, consideration should be given to the distance between the bottom of the tower and the roof deck, the roof deck construction, and the noise sensitivity of the space below the tower. Concrete roof decks are far superior to metal roof decks for transmission noise control.

When a tower is located very close to a building, consideration should be given to the distance between the tower and nearby windows, orientation and closeness of nearby reflecting surfaces, the orientation of the tower, and the adequacy of the wall transmission loss.

SUGGESTED NOISE SPECIFICATIONS

All cooling towers scheduled below shall have been tested in complete accordance with the latest revision of CTI Code ATC-128, Code for Measurement of Sound from Water-Cooling Towers, *shall not exceed the sound pressure levels listed in Table 16-7 at any load capacity.*

TABLE 16-7
Allowable Cooling Tower Octave-Band Sound Pressure Levels and A-Weighted Sound Levels at 50 ft from Faces of the Tower

	Sound Pressure Level dB Octave-Band Center Frequency in Hz								
	(dBA) A-Weighted Sound Level	63	125	250	500	1000	2000	4000	8000
Top									
Back									
End									
End									
Air Inlet									

REFERENCES

ASHRAE. 1995. *1995 ASHRAE handbook—Applications*, p. 43.35. Atlanta: American Society of Heating, Refrigerating and Air-Conditioning Engineers, Inc.

BAC. 1971. The noise of cooling towers. *BAC Engineering Manual 251*. Baltimore Air Coil.

CTI. 1981. *CTI code ATC-128, Code for measurement of sound from water-cooling tower*s. Cooling Tower Institute.

Mason, N. 1966. Mason Industries application notes. ASHRAE lecture.

Miller, L. 1991. Lecture notes for buildings, manufacturing plants, equipment, and products.

Chapter 17
Overview of HVAC Test Procedures

by *Charles Ebbing and Warren Blazier*

SOUND TESTING OF HVAC PRODUCTS

Manufacturers' published information on product sound performance is usually based on specified test setups and/or operating conditions conducted in accordance with ARI, AMCA, ASHRAE, CTI, ASTM, or other industry standards. Table 17-1 presents a guide to the acoustical test standards most often used by the HVAC industry. Representing four generic acoustical test methods, these are

- reverberant-room method for determining sound power level;
- free field above a reflecting plane method for measuring sound pressure level;
- close-in measurement method for measuring sound pressure level;
- acoustic intensity[1] measurements used mainly for diagnostic purposes.

THE REVERBERANT-ROOM METHOD FOR DETERMINING SOUND POWER LEVEL

OVERVIEW

Most HVAC acoustical rating data are determined in reverberant rooms. The HVAC equipment that is normally tested using the reverberation method is identified in Table 17-1 and in Figure 17-1.

1. Acoustic intensity is not currently used as a primary method of rating HVAC products. However, its use is increasing for diagnostic and research measurements.

TABLE 17-1
Guide to Common Sound Standards

HVAC Equipment	Standard	Standard Title	L_w (Power) L_p (Pressure)	Rating Location	Application Std./ Measurement Locations
Air Terminal	ARI 88 ASHRAE 130P	*Air Terminals* (ANSI/ARI 880-89)	L_w	Indoor	ARI 885
Air Diffuser	ARI 890 ASHRAE 70	*Rating of Air Diffusers* and *Air Diffuser Assemblies*	L_w	Indoor	ARI 885
Fan Coil Unit	ARI 350	*Sound Rating of Non-Ducted Indoor Air-Conditioning Equipment*	L_w	Indoor	None
Packaged Air Handler	ARI 260P	*Sound Rating of Ducted Air Moving and Conditioning Equipment*	L_w	Indoor	None
Built Up Air Handler	AMCA 300	*Sound Rating of Ducted Air Moving and Conditioning Equipment*	L_w	Indoor	None
Ventilating Fan	AMCA 300 AMCA 301	*Reverberant Room Method for Sound Testing of Fans; Methods for Calculating Fan Sound Ratings from Laboratory Test Data*	L_w	Indoor	AMCA 302 AMCA 303
Packaged and Year-Round Air-Conditioners (Rooftop)	ARI 260P ARI 370	*Sound Rating of Large Outdoor Refrigeration and Air-Conditioning Equipment*	L_w	Indoor Outdoor	None
Air Cooled Chiller < 10 tons	ARI 270	*Sound Rating of Outdoor Unitary Equipment*	L_w	Outdoor	ARI 275
Air Cooled Chiller > 10 tons	ARI 370	*Sound Rating of Large Outdoor Refrigeration and Air-Conditioning Equipment*	L_w	Outdoor	None

TABLE 17-1 (Continued)
Guide to Common Sound Standards

HVAC Equipment	Standard	Standard Title	L_w (Power) L_p (Pressure)	Rating Location	Application Std./ Measurement Locations
WSHP Water Source Heat Pump	ARI 260P	*Sound Rating of Ducted Air Moving and Conditioning Equipment*	L_w	Indoor	None
Packaged Heat Pump	ARI 260P	*Sound Rating of Ducted Air Moving and Conditioning Equipment*	L_w	Indoor Outdoor	None
Vertical Air Conditioner	ARI 260P	*Sound Rating of Ducted Air Moving and Conditioning Equipment*	L_w	Indoor Outdoor	None
Reciprocating Chiller	ARI 575	*Method of Measuring Machinery Sound within Equipment Rooms*	L_p	Indoor	Avg. Levels at 1 m from Sides of Unit
Screw Chiller	ARI 575	*Method of Measuring Machinery Sound within Equipment Rooms*	L_p	Indoor	Avg. Levels at 1 m from Sides of Unit
Centrifugal Chiller	ARI 575	*Method of Measuring Machinery Sound within Equipment Rooms*	L_p	Indoor	Avg. Levels at 1 m from Sides of Unit
Cooling Tower	CTI Code ATC-128	*Code for Measurement of Sound from Water-Cooling towers*	L_p	Outdoor	Usually Measure at 5 ft and 50 ft on Sides and Top
Centrifugal Water Pump	ANSI/HI 9.1-9.5	*Pumps—General Guidelines*	L_p	Indoor	None
Sound Attenuators	ASTM E-477-96[a] ISO 7235-199[b]	[a]*Standard Test Method for Measuring Acoustical and Air Flow Performance of Duct Liner Materials*	Insertion Loss	N/A	[b]*Acoustics—Measurements Procedures for Ducted Silencers—Insertion Loss, Flow Noise, and Total Pressure Loss*

HVAC Products Tested Using Reverberant Rooms

- Built Up Fans
- Air Terminals
- Exhaust Fans
- Room Fan Coils
- Roof Ventilators
- Air-Handling Units
- Sound Attenuators
- Air-Cooled Water Chillers
- Outdoor Condensing Units
- Packaged Air Conditioners
- Grilles, Registers, and Diffusers

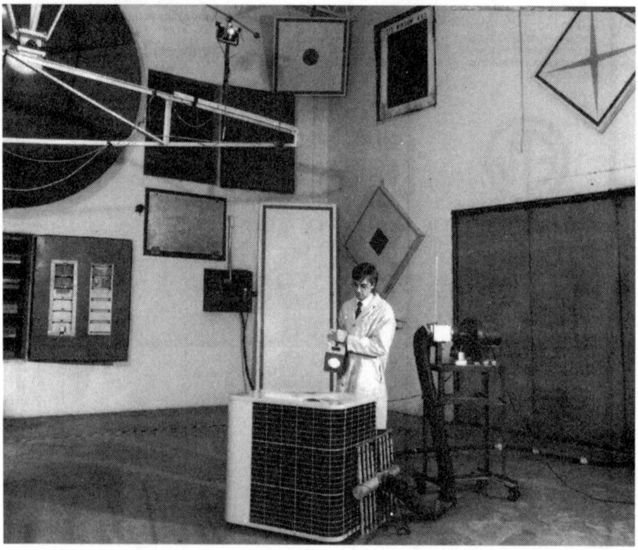

FIGURE 17-1 HVAC equipment normally tested in a reverberant-room facility using various test standards shown in Table 17-1. The example shown is the setup for testing an outdoor air-cooled condensing unit in accordance with ARI 270-84. Ratings are in sound power level, L_W.

Present procedures for testing in reverberant-room facilities are generally applicable only to the frequency range from 100 Hz to 10,000 Hz when measurements are made in one-third octave bands and from 125 Hz to 8,000 Hz when measurements are made in octave bands. ARI[2] has just completed a standard to set qualification requirements for the 63 Hz octave band, and the latest draft of the ISO[3] reverberant-room standard defines the requirements for the 63 Hz octave band testing.

---

2. ARI has recently completed *ARI Standard 280, Requirements for the Qualification of Reverberant Rooms in the 63 Hz Octave Band.* This standard outlines the qualification requirements for the 63 Hz octave band.
3. ISO Draft Standard 3741.

TESTING PACKAGED AIR-HANDLING UNITS

Figures 17-2 through 17-4 show examples of the typical setup for separately determining the sound power level of the discharge, inlet, and casing radiated noise of packaged air-handling units using ARI Standard 260-P.

Testing for Discharge Sound

Figure 17-2 illustrates the test setup for measuring discharge noise. The equipment is installed outside the test room, and the discharge side is connected to the reverberant room. The length of discharge duct used in making this connection is typically equal to 2.5 equivalent duct diameters, which is the same length that would typically be used to determine fan air performance. Relief ducts between the rooms must be used to avoid catastrophically overpressurizing the rooms.[4] The operating characteristics of the fan such as airflow, static pressure, speed, and brake horsepower are usually measured at the same time the fan sound power level data are obtained. This permits the correlation of the measured sound data with the point of operation on the fan curve. Care is also taken to avoid flanking noise problems associated with inadequate vibration isolation between the test unit and the testing facility.

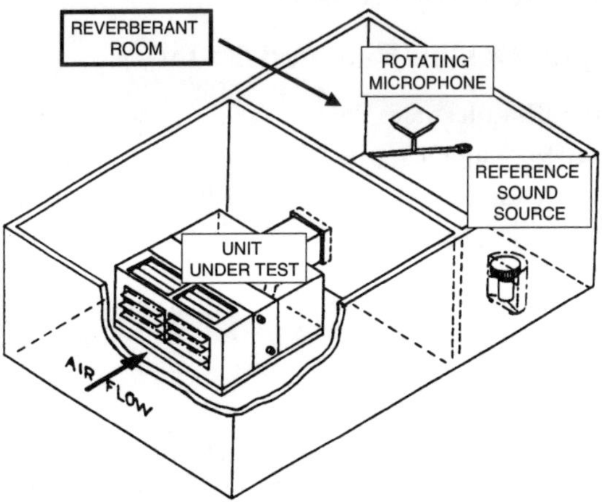

FIGURE 17-2 Testing for discharge sound.

---

4. The reverberant room construction must be capable of safely withstanding the room pressurization necessary to operate the unit at the required static pressure.

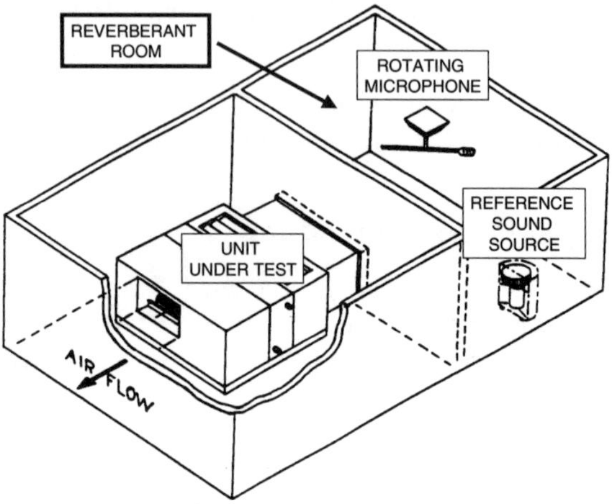

FIGURE 17-3 Testing for inlet sound.

Testing for Inlet Sound

Figure 17-3 illustrates the test setup for measuring inlet noise. The unit is located outside the test room and the inlet side is connected from the reverberant room to the room in which the fan is located. An acoustically lined transfer relief duct is connected between the two rooms to return the air to the fan and avoid overpressurization of the reverberant test room.[5]

Testing for Casing-Radiated Sound

Figure 17-4 illustrates the test setup for measuring casing-radiated sound.[6] The unit is located inside the reverberant room, and the supply and return air are ducted out of the test room. Heavy-gage, stiffened, and lagged ductwork is used to control the sound radiation from the inlet and discharge ductwork within the test room. In this way, only the sound radiated by the casing of the unit is measured.

---

5. A low-resistance transfer duct into the inlet room is also necessary to avoid artificial loading of the inlet side of the unit, thus distorting fan performance and noise measurements. Unit loading is often controlled by a variable resistance in the relief exhaust duct from the discharge room.
6. The accepted term "casing-radiated" sound may be a bit misleading to some readers. This is the sound radiating from the panels or external surfaces of the air handler.

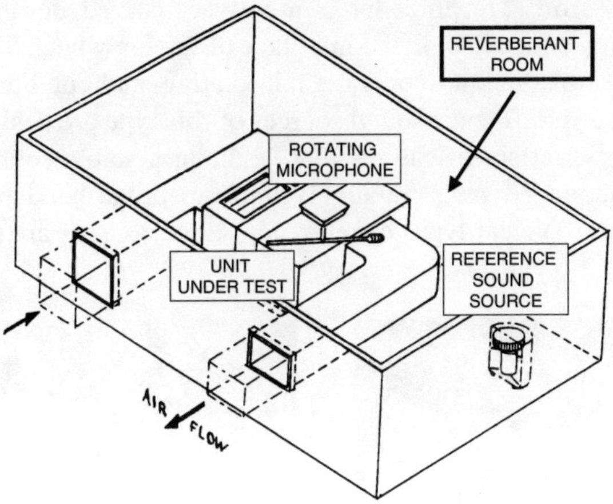

FIGURE 17-4 Testing for casing-radiated sound.

Test Data on Low-Frequency Sound

Current standards for testing in a reverberant room specify measurements down to only 100 Hz. The meaningful determination of sound power level in the octave bands below 63 Hz requires a reverberation room that is substantially larger than 10,000 ft^3. Thus, most manufacturers' sound power level information does not include data at these frequencies because of the prohibitive costs of construction and the difficulties encountered in qualifying the performance of the test room to the tolerances permitted by present standards.

Low-frequency field application data may differ considerably for the installed systems because problems arise from poor aerodynamic design practices in connected ductwork and/or the inappropriate selection of a fan size that cannot cope with system effects. In many cases, the fan becomes unstable and operates inefficiently with much added low-frequency noise in the installed system.

Use of Reference Sound Source in Determining Sound Power Level

Most ARI and AMCA test standards are based on the use of a reference sound source (RSS) in determining the sound power level of a device under test. The most common reference sound source is a small, direct-drive fan wheel that has no volute housing or scroll. The impeller is a forward-curved design with a choke plate installed on the inlet face of the fan wheel. The choke plate causes the fan to operate in a rotating-stall condition that is very noisy. Reference sound sources of this type are designed and built to strict specifications that result in a stable sound power level output having a relatively uniform broad-band frequency spectrum. Typical types of reference sound sources are shown in Figure 17-5 and 17-6.

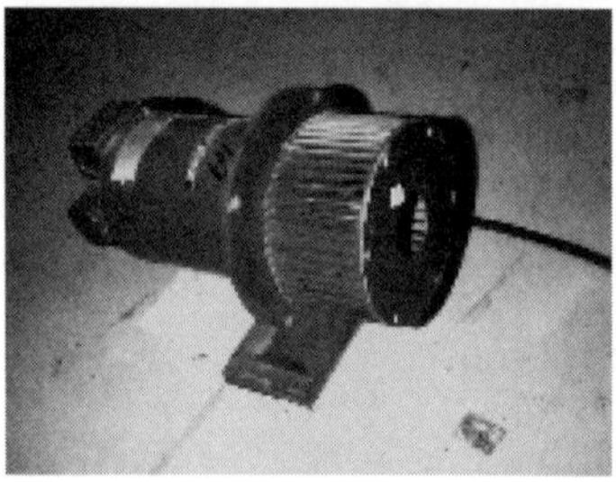

FIGURE 17-5 Horizontal axis reference sound source.

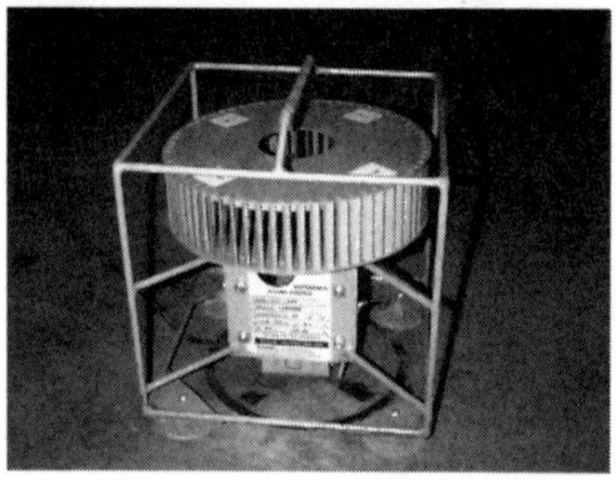

FIGURE 17-6 Vertical axis reference sound source.

However, because of the production of a pure-tone component in the rotating-stall mode of operation, the fan rotational speed determines the lowest frequency at which the unit can be used as a reference sound source. In general, a 3600 rpm unit should not be used below the 125 Hz octave band; an 1800 rpm unit should not be used below the 63 Hz octave band.

To determine the sound power level spectrum of an unknown source, sound pressure level measurements are first made in the reverberant room with the reference sound source operating. Then, the reference source is turned off and similar measurements are made with the HVAC equipment under test in operation. Because the sound power level spectrum of the reference source is known, the measured differences in sound pressure level between the reference source and unknown source correspond to differences in sound power level between the two. Thus, the sound power level of the unknown source can be indirectly determined by adding these differences to the known sound power level of the reference source. This procedure for determining sound power level is known as the *substitution* or *comparison* method.

FREE FIELD ABOVE A REFLECTING PLANE METHOD[7] FOR MEASUREMENT OF SOUND PRESSURE LEVEL

Essentially free-field[8] sound measurement techniques depend upon being able to measure the sound pressure levels directly radiated by the equipment under test without contamination from any sidewall- or ceiling-reflected energy. This is accomplished by either measuring outdoors with the equipment installed on a large paved area or in a hemianechoic[9] room that has highly absorbent sidewalls and ceiling. In either configuration, the accuracy of the method depends upon how closely the measuring space approximates a free-field condition without significant reflections from any surface other than the floor. Large outdoor equipment, such as cooling towers, are typically measured per CTI Code ATC-128 when installed on a large outdoor paved area. As shown in Figure 17-7, sound pressure level measurements are made at fixed distances from the sides

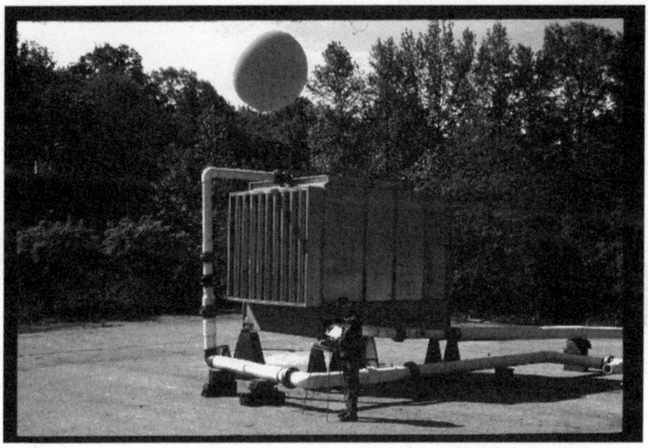

FIGURE 17-7 Measurement of sound pressure level, L_W, from a cooling tower in a free field above a reflecting plane in accordance with CTI Code ATC-128.

7. An essentially free field above a reflecting plane means that there are no significant reflective surfaces close to the source except for the reflective surface on which it rests.
8. Testing rooms that have no significant reflecting surfaces are called free-field or anechoic rooms. They are mainly used for research purposes in the HVAC industry.
9. These test spaces require nonreflective wedges or panels on the walls and ceiling, and the properties of these surfaces determine the lowest frequency that can be accurately measured.

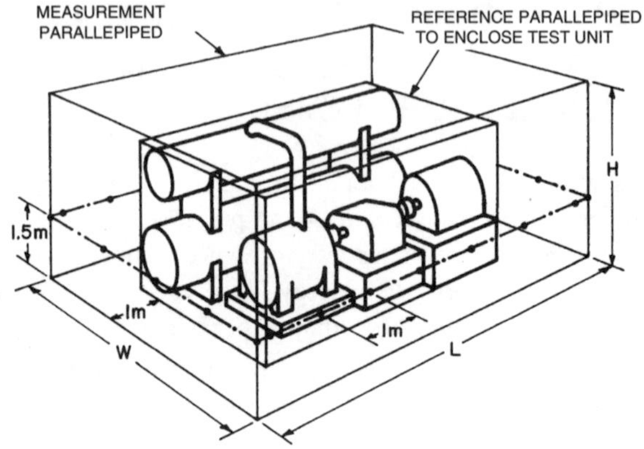

FIGURE 17-8 Measurement of sound pressure level, L_p, from a water-cooled chiller using the close-in method in accordance with ARI Standard 575.

and top of the unit. Sound power levels can also be determined from this data by the method described in Chapter 16.

"CLOSE-IN" METHOD FOR MEASURING SOUND PRESSURE LEVELS

Sound pressure levels radiated by water chillers are measured per ARI Standard 575 at close-in distances of 1 m from the chiller surfaces and at 1.5 m above the floor. ARI 575 does not specify that the measurements be conducted in a free field above reflecting plane environment, but most manufacturers measure in either large rooms or outdoors, which are essentially free field. Chapter 15 discusses the effect of mechanical equipment room size on the data, when the measurements are made indoors.

SOUND INTENSITY METHOD FOR MEASURING SOUND POWER LEVEL

Recent advances in acoustical instrumentation now permit the direct measurement of sound power level.[10] This technique is largely used for research purposes and is seldom used for product rating. This may change over time as technology improves.

10. ANSI Standard S1.12 or ISO 9614-1.

By measuring the sound intensity with a two-channel probe over a surface surrounding a sound source, the sound power radiated by the source can be measured. One advantage of this method is that, with few limitations, sound power measurements can be made in the presence of background noise and in ordinary rooms, thereby eliminating the need for a special testing environment. A second advantage is that, by measuring sound intensity in the close-in area around a sound source, information on local sound directivity[11] can be obtained, which is not possible when using the reverberant-room substitution test method. This can be particularly useful in the noise reduction aspects of product development. One disadvantage is that sound intensity measurements are sensitive to local air velocities that may be present in the vicinity of the probes and that introduce errors if the velocity is greater than 400 fpm to 500 fpm.

Sound intensity measurement procedures are still experimental and require significant expertise to obtain meaningful and reliable rating data.

STANDARDS FOR TESTING DUCT SILENCERS

The present standards used for testing dissipative and reactive silencers are ASTM E477-96 in North America and ISO 7235-1991 elsewhere. There currently are no standard test methods available to test the performance of active silencers. Figure 17-9 illustrates a typical test setup for determining a silencer's insertion loss, pressure drop, and airflow-generated noise using ASTM-E477-96.

To measure insertion loss, two separate measurements must be made. The sound pressure level in the reverberation room is measured while noise generated by loudspeakers enters the room through a length of straight empty duct. The sound pressure is measured again after a section of the empty duct has been replaced with the silencer. The insertion loss is the difference between the two measured levels.

Silencer pressure drop is obtained by measuring the total pressure 5 diameters downstream of the silencer and subtracting it from the total pressure measured 2.5 diameters upstream. To ensure streamlined airflow for accurate measurements, a minimum of five

---

11. Sound directivity enables one to identify the noisiest radiating parts or surfaces of the source and the noisiest radiating directions. See Figures 16-2 and 16-3 for an example.

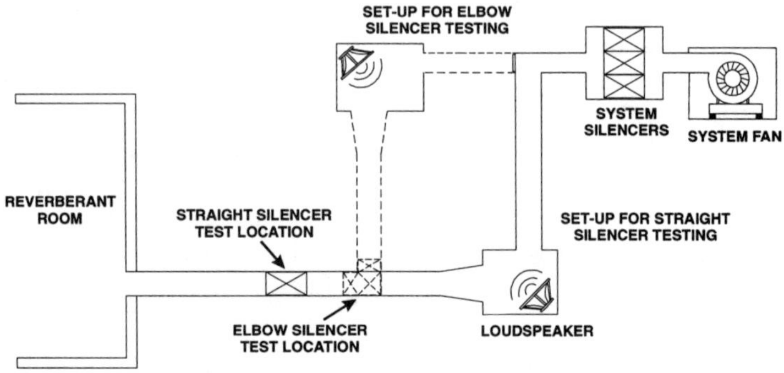

FIGURE 17-9 Typical silencer testing arrangement.

diameters of straight duct on the inlet side of the silencer and ten diameters of straight duct following the discharge of the silencer are required.

The airflow-generated sound power levels are calculated from measured sound pressure levels in the reverberation room when originally quiet air passes through the system with the silencer installed.

The substitution method is used to calculate the sound power levels. End reflection corrections per AMCA must be added to the sound power based on the termination cross section of the system duct at the reverberation room wall. Current standards do not account for possible acoustic losses from the system duct between the silencer and the reverberation room.

Variations of ±3 dB in insertion loss values can be expected down to 63 Hz although there are presently no ANSI or ISO standards to qualify reverberation chambers below 100 Hz. Generated noise testing produces greater variation. A recent round-robin showed five different laboratories reporting ±3 dB to ± 6 dB over the octave-band frequency range of 125 Hz to 8000 Hz when testing for generated noise according to ASTM E-477-96. Accurate data were not available below 100 Hz. Similar round-robins are not known to the authors to be held for the ISO 7235-1991 standard.

When evaluating elbow and transition silencer insertion loss and pressure drop test data, it is critical to evaluate the reference empty duct section. Elbow silencers can be tested according to the ISO 7235-1991 standard using an empty duct fitting as the reference. The ASTM E-477-96 standard does not yet include provisions for testing elbow silencers. Manufacturers could use a straight length or a sheet metal elbow (mitered or radiused, with or without turning vanes) as the reference empty duct. Each case will yield varying insertion loss data for the same silencer. Therefore, for elbow and transition silencers, a description of the substituted duct element must be reported along with any performance data.

While many similarities exist, the ASTM and ISO standards produce differing results because of variations in loudspeaker location orientation, duct termination conditions, and computation methodology.

VARIABILITY OF TEST DATA

Whether manufacturers' ratings are approached in a typical field application depends mainly upon the details of product application, as has been documented in the previous chapters of this book.

Whatever method of test used, variation and uncertainty are expected due to different laboratories having different size or instrumentation. Tables in each product chapter in this book give estimates of the likely uncertainties involved.

REFERENCES

ASHRAE. 1995. *1995 ASHRAE handbook—Applications*, p. 43.19. Atlanta: American Society of Heating, Refrigerating and Air-Conditioning Engineers, Inc.